✓ 14.95

‖‖‖‖‖‖‖‖‖‖‖‖‖‖‖‖‖‖‖‖‖

W9-BNA-294

SWEET
GRAPES

WOMEN'S COLLEGE HOSPITAL
WOMEN'S HEALTH CENTRE
THE RESOURCE CENTRE

SWEET
GRAPES

How to Stop Being Infertile
And Start Living Again

Jean W. Carter and Michael Carter

Perspectives Press
Indianapolis, IN

WP
570
C37
1989
00002326

copyright © 1989 by Michael Carter and Jean W. Carter

All rights reserved. No part of this book may be reproduced in any manner or form whatsoever, electrical or mechanical, including photocopying, recording, or by information storage and retrieval systems without written permission except in the case of brief quotations embodied in critical articles and reviews. For information, address the publisher at:

Perspectives Press
P.O. Box 90318
Indianapolis, Indiana 46290-0318

Manufactured in the United States of America
ISBN # 0-9609504-9-4 (hardcover); # 0-944934-01-3 (paperback)

Library of Congress Cataloging-in-Publication Data

Carter, Jean W., 1951-
 Sweet grapes : how to stop being infertile and start living again / Jean W. Carter and Michael Carter.
  p.   cm.
 Bibliography: p.
 ISBN 0-9609504-9-4 : $13.95.
 ISBN 0-944934-01-3 (pbk.) : $8.95
 1. Infertility--Popular works. 2. Childlessness.
I. Carter, Michael, 1950- . II. Title.
RC889.C37 1989
155.9'16--dc20   89-34135
                                                   CIP

necessarily your infertility. The way to resolve your infertility is by becoming no longer infertile—before you adopt! Not being infertile frees you to adopt a child because you *want* to adopt a child. Without this kind of freedom, Plumez says, the adopted child is likely to be "second best," only a substitute for your biological child. We have a special name for this state of not being infertile so that you have the opportunity to adopt—being open to adoption.

The problem is that many couples who cannot be fertile continue to live their lives as infertile (as opposed to no longer infertile). If they remain childless, they define their lives in terms of the child they will never have. And even if they adopt they continue to define their lives by the *biological* child they don't have and continue to hope for. We say that there is another way. No longer being infertile focuses not on the loss but on the possibility for gain. It changes childless into childfree and adoption as second best into adoption as first best.

So childfree and open to adoption are both ways of becoming no longer infertile. We have discovered, though, that a lot of people see them as opposing options. Some think that deciding not to adopt means that they are automatically childfree, and others perceive of childfree as anti-adoption. We will talk in greater length about these misconceptions later, but let's consider them briefly now.

Living childfree and being open to adoption have a lot more in common than most people believe. First of all, both should be the result of a choice. If you think of adoption as simply the next logical step in the infertility process, then perhaps you haven't put your infertility behind you. And if childfree means simply that you don't want to adopt, perhaps you also have not been able to break out of your infertility. Indeed, being open to adoption may be considered "biological childfree." If childfree is living with the advantages of not having children, then "biological childfree" might be defined as living with the advantage of not having a biological child—that advantage is that you can adopt a child and share in the experience of an adoptive family.

Also, the decision to adopt and the decision to live childfree are both *positive* choices. And a positive choice cannot be the result of a rejection of something else. A childfree life cannot be founded on a rejection of adoption. People who adopt should not perceive of childfree as a threat. And people who are childfree should not perceive of adoption as a threat. They should both be choices *in favor* of something, not against.

Finally, they are both an affirmation of a way of life, one an affirmation of a life without children and the other an affirmation of a life with an adopted child. Both depend on this affirmation. In both cases the affirmation leads to something good. In one case it is the possibility of a satisfying life without children, in the other case it is the ability to adopt a child with a different configuration of genes and love him or her as your own.

Childfree and adoption are not opposing positions. They are both indications that you are ready to get on with your life as no longer infertile.

3. The Focus of This Book

The main subject of this book is the childfree way of becoming no longer infertile. We have chosen this focus for several reasons. One is that we are childfree. That is the way we have made the transition from infertile to no longer infertile, so that is what we are most experienced with. Another reason is that childfree is so widely misunderstood. We feel that a large part of our task is to help people understand what childfree is and how to become childfree, an attempt to reduce the confusion about it.

A third reason is that of all the couples who cannot conceive, only about 25% of them even try to adopt (as reported in 1980), a percentage that seems to be dropping. And our experience tells us that many of the people who don't adopt are still focused on the child they don't have; they are still infertile. Because this is such a large group, we wanted to address the potential they possess for living childfree.

Fourth, there are dozens of books on infertility and adoption, but we haven't found another one specifically on living childfree after infertility. We think that this subject demands special considerations that don't appear in books aimed at the voluntarily childfree. And finally, we believe it's important for couples who are considering adoption at least to understand the childfree alternative. We see ourselves as childfree advocates, but we certainly don't recommend it for everyone; however, we do think that adoption should be a choice that a couple makes, and part of making a choice is to consider the other possibilities. Otherwise it's not really a choice.

Though the focus of this book is mainly on childfree, we are also concerned with the larger issue of no longer being infertile. This means that much of what we say about childfree is also relevant to adoption, particularly Chapters Three, Four, Five, and Eight. In Chapter Three we discuss the potential that we all possess for turning the loss of infertility into a gain. In Chapters Four and Five we talk about the crucial role that choice plays in achieving that potential. And in Chapter Eight, we apply what we have said about no longer being infertile specifically to the diverse kinds of adoption.

But even though our emphasis is on no longer being infertile, it's possible to find an even broader focus in this book. It also has implications for other major losses that occur in our lives. It is a book about taking a major loss and finding in it the opportunity for a major gain. Indeed, this may be the greatest lesson of all because it gives us hope that all loss—such as losing a job, living with a less-than-perfect child, getting a divorce, or even dying—offers the potential for growth.

Jean Tells Our Story

We never talked much about children before we got married. They were a part of our distant future and we simply expected them to come, one of life's givens, as inevitable as aging. Our immediate concerns at that time were marriage, school, and  managing two careers, in that order. But when we did mention children it was always in sentences that began, "When we have children . . ."

We got married when I was beginning my third year of medical school and Mike was beginning graduate school in English, so it was easy—necessary even—to postpone children. Five years later, though, as I began to hear the biological clock ticking louder and louder and with the physically most demanding years of a residency in obstetrics and gynecology behind me, we began to talk seriously about having children. To our surprise, we discovered that we felt some ambivalence about the issue. After concentrating so long on our professional lives, we found some self doubt in the face of this new responsibility. It wasn't that either one of us expressed any strong desire *not* to have children, but we both recognized the seriousness of the step. It wasn't long, though, before we decided yes, we want to have children. We wanted to affirm our belief in life and our love for each other. We may have begun with ambivalence, but we discovered that our desire for children was no less strong for it; in fact, wrestling with the issue may have strengthened that desire. We wanted a child.

The story of the next three years is familiar to most couples who have faced problems with their fertility. At first we felt foolish at the disappointment we felt when my period would come. We knew that it takes time. But when a few months became a year, we began to fear that something might be wrong. As an obstetrician I knew all the advice that doctors gave for getting pregnant, so even before we became infertility patients the basal temperature thermometer became a bedside fixture and sex became a routine dictated by the calendar.

When even these efforts produced no baby, we decided that the time had come to seek help from an infertility specialist. The fact that I was an OB/GYN resident made our infertility workup both easier and more difficult than most couples'. Because I worked with infertility patients myself, I knew where to go for the best care and had easy access to the doctors who could give me that care. But there were disadvantages, too. I had delayed going to see a doctor because of a professional pride that led me to believe that I could solve the problem myself. I also knew all about the difficult tests and procedures that come with an infertility workup and treatment. The worst thing about being an insider, though, was that I was often treated more like a colleague than a patient. I found myself wanting more specific explanations, more counseling, more *comforting.* And worse yet, I was the one who had to translate all the medical jargon into laymen's terms for Mike, outlining for him the risks and alternatives for tests and treatments. It was hard to do that objectively, particularly when *I* was the one being discussed!

Physician heal thyself had its humorous side, too. At one point in our workup we were asked to obtain some cervical mucus and mail it in dry ice to a lab in Michigan. Getting the dry ice and packaging was no problem, but getting the mucus was. At that time I was beginning private practice and was unwilling (for reasons of modesty?) to ask my new partners to get the mucus for me. So Mike and I decided to do it ourselves. When the right time of the month came around, we sneaked into my office late at night after everyone, including the janitor, had gone. We felt like comic thieves in a movie and even jumped like frightened deer when a water cooler abruptly turned on. I got into the stirrups and with a hand mirror directed Mike through his first gynecological exam. Mike, who doesn't even like for me to *talk* about what I do, was sweating awfully under the hot lights he was using to see through the speculum as I called out what to do: "It's that round thing in the middle. No, over there. Yes, that's it. Now take the . . ." We never did get the mucus but at least Mike no longer suffers from professional envy.

Early in our workup we felt relieved when each test came back normal. But as more and more tests showed normal results, I began to worry. I knew that in about 10% of infertile couples no cause for the problem is ever found. I also knew that this group has one of the poorest chances for ever achieving a pregnancy. You can't fix what isn't broken.

By the third year of trying to conceive, we were being offered very little encouragement by the specialists. And as our hopes for a biological child dimmed, we began to grieve in earnest. Each menstrual period touched off rage and depression. Every baby I saw made me acutely aware of the emptiness in my belly and in my arms. But the worst times were when a friend or relative would announce a pregnancy. And it seemed that all my friends from high school and college were having babies and sending baby pictures. The biggest depression came when Mike's sister-in-law got pregnant, the first grandchild in Mike's family. He kept the news to himself until he thought the time was right for a storm to break—and it did.

The full force of our infertility hit home, literally, when we made a special trip to tell our parents that we would probably not be giving them grandchildren. I found out several years later that Mike's parents thought we were coming to announce that we were pregnant, since we had let on some time before that we were trying. So it was even more remarkable that they kept what must have been a great disappointment from showing. We all cried a little, and for the first time in a long time, Mike and I felt absolutely accepted—even though we were infertile.

The next day, however, has become famous in our family lore. Mike and I went to church with his parents and, wouldn't you know it, they had scheduled an infant baptism. At Mike's church, baptisms are a big deal. The minister takes the baby in his arms and carries her around the sanctuary, introducing the baby to her new church family. But on that occasion, this loving ritual was only a reminder of a blessing that I couldn't have. I found myself crying. And I don't mean just a few discrete tears but boohooing. To make matters worse, we were sitting right in the front of the church, so I couldn't just ease out. I sat there and cried—with people passing Kleenex and handkerchiefs to me —till the parents finally took their beautiful baby away.

Most infertile people find that they are able to avoid babies and baby talk and occasions like that baptism. But not an obstetrician. I was never far from a swollen belly or a proud father. But even worse were those unhappily pregnant women wanting referral to an abortion center. And I found that I shared the pain of my infertility patients much too deeply. Looking back on it now, though, I can see that this daily dose of pain was actually a blessing. I knew I couldn't go on living that way. Something had to change. I had to get either a new job or a new attitude.

That new attitude started to blossom in the spring of 1983 when Mike and I attended a day-long workshop for infertile people on the campus of Purdue University, sponsored by the Indiana chapter of RESOLVE, the national infertility support organization. I pushed and persuaded a reluctant Mike to go with me to the meeting, together as an infertile couple rather than by myself as a gynecologist—in disguise, so to speak. In fact, I remember promising to do the dishes for two weeks if he would go. He gave in to the bribery and agreed to go but not to enjoy it. Going was enough for me.

When we arrived at the workshop, Mike tried his best to become invisible in the way that husbands sometimes do at gatherings. I had a professional excuse for being there, but for him it was an open admission of failure, as if his masculinity had become tied up in his fertility. He joked that his name tag should read, "Hi, I'm Mike Carter and I'm infertile." But as the day went on, he became involved and interested—and visible. He discovered that there were men there, some of whom he knew but hadn't realized they were also infertile. But best of all he discovered our infertility was a problem that we shared with many other nice, normal people and was nothing to be ashamed of.

The workshop consisted of a smorgasbord of hour-long discussions on topics of medical, emotional, and marital issues related to infertility, such as advice on pursuing adoption, scientific talks on the causes of infertility, and presentations about new treatments. One title, "Childless to Childfree," intrigued us, so we both attended. In retrospect, the couple who gave the talk was still carrying some anger and bitterness, but they were in the process of forging a new life for themselves. This was the first time that the concept of living childfree had even occurred to us.

We both feel that this seminar was a major turning point for us. We didn't find an answer there, but it started us talking in a way we never had talked before. It was as though a taboo had been lifted. The main thing was that these were issues that *could* be talked about and dealt with as we did with other problems. After the meeting was over, I remember walking back and forth in the late evening sun over what seemed like miles of brick sidewalks on the Purdue campus—talking and talking.

Nothing was solved that day, but it did touch off months of discussing, negotiating, questioning, arguing—all of which allowed us to learn more about ourselves and each other. The wonderful thing was that we *were* talking. We were beginning to feel that we had some control over our lives again. We stopped seeing ourselves as victims, helpless in the hands of fate. There were decisions that we could make. The way we saw it, our choices were these: to keep on hoping and trying after medical means had been exhausted, to adopt, or to live childfree.

There was only one more test being offered to us, a diagnostic laparoscopy in which my pelvic organs would be examined in a minor surgical procedure under general anesthesia to look for any other physical causes of our infertility, such as endometriosis. We agreed to go ahead with that step, but in the weeks before it, we played "what if." What if, once again, nothing abnormal were found? What would we do? We knew that if the laparoscopy turned up nothing treatable then we were finished with medical help. We also knew that we weren't going to keep riding the 28-day cycle of hope, failure, and despair.

That left adoption to consider. This question was much more difficult for us to answer. We went through times of strong feelings both ways, usually out of sync with each other. We finally came to the mutual conclusion that adoption was not for us. Our choice was based on an unequal mixture of logical, realistic concerns—such as the very short supply of adoptable babies and doubts about our suitability as adoptive parents—and completely irrational considerations. The important thing is that we talked about it and kept talking. Neither one of us allowed the other to play the role of dictator. And as we talked we were able to bring to light some deep-seated fears, doubts, and needs that may have nothing to do with logic or the way life really is but are no less strong for that.

So we began to ask ourselves some questions. Could we be happy without children? Could we accept a life as nonparents? Could be choose it and affirm it? Could we change childless to childfree?

Soon, in the fall of 1983, it was time for the laparoscopy, and once again my being a doctor was both an advantage and a disadvantage. I was able to get the surgery done by the best person in the area, but I had done the procedure many times myself and knew precisely what to expect. Sometimes a little ignorance can be relatively blissful. My position as doctor-patient became especially pronounced as Mike and I were waiting nervously before the operation in the pre-surgical holding area. First an I.V. technician came in to put the preoperative I.V. line into my vein, but when the nurse introduced me as a doctor he blanched slightly and eased out of the room. Then the resident came in and the same thing happened. Then the chief resident. I thought for a moment that I was going to have to talk an unwilling Mike through another medical procedure, but finally the attending anesthesiologist came to do the job. Fortunately he had no trouble.

I woke up in the recovery room with the surgeon's face blurring in and out saying, "Everything looks just fine in there." My immediate reaction was relief that I was well and would not have to undergo treatment for endometriosis. My second reaction was relief also, but for a different reason. I knew that I was getting off the infertility roller coaster at last. All of our talking had led us to the place where we could make a choice to live childfree. Of course, there was still some final grieving to do. Hope is hard to give up, even when it has become more painful than helpful.

Finally, there came a day that winter when after so many weeks of talking about living childfree, we finally decided to choose it—to take it and live it. We didn't know exactly what it meant, but we were willing to figure it out day by day and build the rest of our lives on it. The most important thing was that we realized that we *did* have a choice. We could be child*less*, defining our lives by what we lack, or we could be child*free*, affirming the potential gain that comes of living without children. We chose the latter.

Things really did begin to get better from that moment as one small part of our lives after another underwent redefinition. The future nursery turned into a music room. The dolls we had been saving for our daughters were set aside for our nieces. The money we had been putting away as a college fund became our opportunity to travel. After dozens of these little transformations, we realized that we had made a major change in our lives. Instead of being unsuccessful parents-to-be, we were very successful nonparents. Failure was no longer the major theme of our lives.

Neither one of us had realized how much of our lives had been consumed by infertility until we chose to live childfree. Suddenly we found energy for doing things. I began quilting and Mike began to work in earnest on his dissertation. We became more active in community and church activities. We felt that once more we were in control of our lives—and could do something with them.

There were two more important milestones on our road to a childfree resolution. The first occurred almost a year after we made our decision. One Friday night, at the beginning of what promised to be a romantic weekend, I came home with a package of contraceptive sponges. And Mike's reaction was, "Yes, that's a good idea." We seemed to have arrived together at the point where it was time to exert that final bit of control over our reproductive lives. We know that Mother Nature's sense of humor is just bizarre enough to wait until my fortieth birthday to grant the wish we long ago stopped wishing for, and we didn't intend to let her do that. We also realized that even though we had decided to live childfree, there was always that little bit of hope each month that I would not get my period, enough hope, though, to hurt. Contraception was our declaration of independence from the cycle of hope and despair and for us the final step in being childfree.

The second milestone came shortly after the first, when

we were asked to speak to a RESOLVE chapter meeting about the childfree alternative. Preparing for the talk forced us to go back over our journey, step by step, which was a painful process. But it was only through that process that we began to understand what we had done, and we discovered that it seemed to make sense. We realized that choosing to live childfree is just as "successful" a way of resolving an infertility crisis as having a biological child or adopting. It is not a failure or a resignation to fate; instead, it is an affirmation of who we are and of our ability to live full, productive, happy lives because of who we are. We discovered that we don't need children to be a family.

We also discovered that this is a very difficult concept, especially for people who have spent much of their recent lives trying to have children. It sounds like giving up or taking second best. One woman asked us, in a rather accusing tone, whether if we were offered an easy medical cure for our infertility problem, wouldn't we take the cure and have children? We both responded without hesitation that we wouldn't. That part of our lives is over. We like who we are now, and our plans for our lives do not include children of our own.

But our lives do include other children. One especially pleasing consequence of our choice to live childfree was that children came back into our lives. We had avoided them as much as possible during the struggle with our infertility because of the pain they caused us. But we found ourselves opening our hearts to children once again. We no longer perceive them as reminders of what we don't have, ready evidence of our inadequacy. At this writing, we are enriched by two god-daughters, three nieces, and two nephews. And we love birthday parties.

This transformation has probably meant more to me than to Mike. One of the reasons I became an obstetrician was the joy of watching a mother's belly grow and of bringing a baby into a loving family. When I was infertile, though, all this changed. The joy was replaced by jealousy and pain; the baby business was no longer a happy one for me. Deciding to live childfree brought the joy back. I no longer look at pregnant women as a threat. I still may cry a little at a birth but it's not because of jealousy any more. Now the tears are once again tears of happiness for the baby and for its mother and father. This baby and their love for this baby are *my* hope for the future, *my* legacy, *my* joy.

What It Means to Live Childfree

What's in a name? that which we call a rose
By any other name would smell as sweet.

—Shakespeare

Childfree is one of those awkward words that has no established meaning. You won't find it in the dictionary because it hasn't been entered into common usage in our language. So it wanders around, meaning different things to different people. What we would like to do in this chapter is to try pinning it down by presenting our concept of childfree.

In *Romeo and Juliet*, Juliet asked the famous question, "What's in a name?" She was talking about the family names that separated her family from Romeo's, but what she also wanted to know was whether names of things have any real significance. We could ask the same question about a name like *childfree*. Is there any real difference between it and child*less*, that word that infertile people hate to use because of its awful finality? Isn't childfree simply a pleasant way of saying that you have failed to have a baby?

For us, childfree *is* significantly different from childless. Childfree is a word that describes the positive potential in living without children. It is a hopeful word that points to one way of finding a happy ending to infertility. We are sympathetic, however, to people who may at first be put off by the term, especially infertile people who are in the midst of an infertility workup and treatment. We know how that feels and we understand how childfree may have hurtful connotations of not wanting children, not liking children and seeking to be free of them. We hope that in this book we can change those connotations.

Juliet, of course, learned the hard way that there is a lot in a name. But the power in a name comes not so much from the name itself but from what it does. For us, the important thing about childfree is that it offers us one way to stop being infertile. In this chapter we will look a little more closely at what that means.

1. Childfree Means Changing Negative into Positive

Childfree. The word itself implies that living without children can be a positive experience. The alternative, of course, is child*less*, with its connotations of something missing from your life, an incompleteness. Childfree is the positive side of this coin. It means living without children, but living without them in a positive way. It suggests a completeness that you can achieve even without children.

Some people, however, have seen something different in childfree. They say that childfree is a word that should be used only for those who *never wanted* to have children. Those who are infertile, they say, cannot be childfree. According to this view, infertile people should think of themselves as child*less*, thus separating themselves from the voluntarily childfree. The word childless becomes a sort of red badge of infertility that only a few war weary veterans can wear, leaving childfree to those who not only never made it to the front but were not even called into service. This concept of childfree carries with it the unsavory connotations of not liking children and glad to be free of them, difficult connotations for people who have sacrificed so much in *trying to have* children.

We certainly understand how these people could derive such negative connotations from childfree, and we respect their need to see themselves as distinct from those who haven't been through what they have. For us, however, and for many others who have battled infertility, what we crave is not a red badge of infertility but a peace that allows us to live in harmony with ourselves. We want to put our infertility behind us and get on with our lives in as positive a way as possible. This is what childfree offers.

2. Childfree Means Taking Advantage of the Advantages

For us, the difference between childless and childfree is not just a superficial play of semantics. Childfree is not just putting the veneer of a happy face over a rotten situation. Instead, it means learning to see yourself and your life without children in a positive light. And a big part of this is embracing the benefits of living without children.

Some of these benefits are obvious, and on a bad day any parent could help add to the list. People typically think of such things as freedom to go out, to travel, to do things spontaneously. They also point to added resources of time, energy, and creativity. And, of course, if your career is important to you, it can be a great luxury to go out the door in the morning without feeling torn in two, or to stay late without feeling guilty. Even if work isn't fun or fulfilling, the after-work hours can be spent on something that is. Or a career that's not working out can be scrapped while you go back to school or try something new.

Another obvious advantage is financial. Experts estimate that it will cost around $140,000 to raise and educate one child. This does not even count the loss of the mother's earnings and career advancement. For many couples this can mean the difference between struggling and living comfortably. Not having to worry about the financial burden of raising children has given us much more flexibility with our careers than our friends who have children, allowing us to make a highly satisfying but unprofitable career move which we might not have made if we had been thinking about orthodontia and college tuition. Because we were childfree, we could take advantage of the freedom to make *less* money.

One of our correspondants, Sally, reports that she is realizing some of the financial benefits of living childfree: "I am excited about the freedom both in time and money that childfree living offers. My husband and I are now planning trips and possibly buying a country home—which we could never afford if we had a child."

There are other benefits of living childfree that are less tangible. The energy that is absorbed by children can be turned to other contributions in the church or synagogue, the community, or the arts. You can also invest this energy in your relationship with each other. Couples with children tend to go through long periods when they are too busy meeting the children's needs to take care of each other. They may be unable to keep in close contact as they grow and change through the years and often have to go through the process of rediscovering each other after the kids are gone. Some even lose each other and their marriages in the process. Childless couples have the luxury of more time for each other, time to communicate with each other, time for physical closeness without fear of interruption, time to spend on leisure activities together, and time to work together toward common goals.

But there is another side of this coin, too. Some couples may need the extra "elbow room" that being childfree gives. We know some childfree couples who thrive on the independence that not having children brings them. Their marriage is important to them but so is the ability to engage in their separate interests and friends without the obligation for "family" activities that having children demands. Being childfree allows them the mutual independence that they enjoy.

But before you start drawing the wrong conclusion, we want to point out that we know that our focus on the advantages of living childfree might be misinterpreted as selfishness. This is the same reaction we found in a cover story on the voluntarily childless in *Newsweek* a couple of years ago. The article portrayed these couples who had chosen not to have children as shallow and self-absorbed. For instance, one couple claimed as their reason for not having children the fact that they had a white carpet and children would track it up.

This *Newsweek* story expressed the popular opinion that people who choose not to have children must be selfish. But charges of selfishness are difficult to defend for most couples who choose not to have children and are especially ridiculous when leveled at couples who have endured the pain and sacrifices of infertility. When we talk about the benefits of living childfree after infertility, we are by no means trying to claim that there are direct compensations for not having children. There is no equation in which three romantic dinners equal one wet kiss on the cheek. On the other hand, if there *are* some benefits to living without children, why not take advantage of them? This is what childfree couples do. They make the most of their lives with the opportunities offered to them by not having children.

Anne Smith says it well: "In making the childfree decision you shouldn't think of what you don't have, but what you can have. Opportunities will be available to you that you may never have dreamed of, a whole new world will open up to you once you make and accept the decision."

This is not selfishness! On the contrary, it is a sensible approach to life in which you live in the light of the advantages you find. Not in the sense of making the best of a bad situation, which continues to dwell on the negative, but in emphasizing the opportunities, making your life good because it can be good.

3. Childfree Means Taking Control of your Life Again

"I think what really bothers us most about not having children," Susan told us, "was that suddenly we (who had everything planned and our lives under control) had come up against something over which we had no control. Feeling out of control and suddenly at the mercy of others (doctors, adoption agencies, etc.) really got to us!"

For most couples, one of the most excruciating aspects of infertility is the loss of control. Losing control over our reproduction spills over into other parts of our lives. The plans for having children, often carefully plotted, collapse. Sex becomes a routine function and often simply an inconvenience. Work schedules are sacrificed for clinic visits. We take potentially dangerous drugs and treatments that we never would have considered before. In short, our bodies and our lives are no longer our own.

Being childfree enables you to regain control of your life once again because it allows you to create a new identity for yourself—as a person who is no longer infertile. Naomi Pfeffer and Anne Woolit, two British writers, describe this process of creating a new identity as a combination of becoming a new person and rediscovering and reaffirming who you are. In their insightful book, *The Experience of Infertility*, they elaborate on this idea:

> Creating a new identity without children is an important part of asserting control over your

infertility. This involves trying to think beyond children and deciding what you want for yourself ... It involves giving up your desires for a child while not regretting the time you have spent in your quest ... Creating a new identity does not mean abandoning your reasons for wanting a child. Just as those reasons shaped your infertility experience, so they affect the form that your resolution takes. Your new identity can accommodate some of the motives that you had for wanting a child. You need to be able to acknowledge and accept those ideas so you can build upon them, and take their essence into account. It is not a question of giving up ideas which seemed important, or of denying the power they had for you, but of looking for new ways of working on those ideas.

One strategy for creating a new identity is to look back at what life was like before you started to pursue pregnancy. What used to make you happy? What did you look forward to? What was important to you? Of course, you can't go back in time and deny that infertility has changed and shaped you, but you can try to recapture the essence of who you were.

Another strategy is to find new outlets for the motivations that made you want to have children in the first place. If you had a desire to nurture, you can find another way of doing this. We are lucky in that our jobs as a physician and a college teacher give us daily opportunities to help people grow. But people whose jobs don't offer this will need to find another way to build, grow, teach, or develop. The world is hungry for people who have those inclinations and the time to act on them.

If children were to be your immortality, you can find some other way to be remembered after you are gone. We can't all be rich enough to endow a fund or to have our name in brass letters on a building, but we can make enough of a difference while we are here that we will not be soon forgotten. This can mean a work of art, an idea for other thinkers to build on, a generation of third-graders, or even a corner store that will not be the same without us.

Unfortunately, women seem to have more difficulty in

creating a fresh identity for themselves apart from children. They may see themselves as feminine only insofar as they are able to bear and rear children. Or they may see their marriages in the same light—pointless without children. Pfeffer and Woolit address this issue directly and in a way that deserves another long quotation.

> By whatever route you came to the decision to have a child, your self-esteem has been battered by your infertility. Coping and coming to terms with it means coming to see yourself as all right again. Like other women without children, like women who have chosen not to have them, or like older women whose children have grown up, you are a person who can be loved, liked, and lusted after. Children in themselves do not make you any more likeable, womanly, able to relate to other people or productive in other areas of your life. In fact the contrary may be true. Women with children have less time and energy to give to other people and develop interests outside their families.
>
> Relationships based solely on a mutual desire for a child must be rare. It is important to recollect those aspects of each other that you found attractive before the [infertility] investigations started and try to recover old ways of relating to each other; and you need to find new ways too that are not centered around a child or anticipation of a child.
>
> Ultimately all parents have to find an identity beyond parenthood and it may be possible to gain strength by looking at women older than yourself to see how they cope with their loss . . . when their children no longer need their day-to-day care.

Another way that living childfree helps you to take control again is that it encourages you to redefine parts of your life. Redefinition, though, may come gradually. After so many years, giving up some of the hurt is almost like breaking a bad habit. But after you have made the decision to live childfree, a wonderful thing begins to happen. One by one things that were bad become neutral and eventually good. Events that have always been painful come to lose their power over you.

For example, the start of a menstrual period, which had been a monthly signal for a serious crying jag, once again becomes a normal, healthy event. Because childfree means that you have decided to make your life good without children, having your period is a good thing. The change in the menstrual period from failure to success mirrors the change in your life. Failure is no longer its dominant theme, with all other accomplishments overshadowed by the one great non-success at achieving pregnancy. You are no longer a failure as a parent, but a great success an a non-parent.

For us, perhaps the most pleasant effect of the redefinition that comes with being childfree is that we were able to bring children back into our lives. Like so many other infertile couples, we had built walls around ourselves to protect us from the pain associated with other people's children. Birthday parties, christenings, and family holidays had become unendurable because they accentuated our own lack of fertility, our inability to be a part of this child-oriented society. But after we had accepted and embraced our life as it was, we could tear down those walls. It is ironic that it was only when we became childfree that we rediscovered children and could share in our fertile friends' happiness. Now we look forward to birthday parties, we can share in the joy of someone else's birth announcement, and we can enjoy the wonderful chaos that children bring to family events.

The joy of knowing other people's children can go both ways. Wanda observed that "every child deserves a childless aunt and uncle." She remembered her own childless aunt and uncle with a great fondness because when she was a child they made her feel special in a way that, because of her large family, she didn't feel at home. And when she was older, she could tell them things she couldn't tell her parents. Almost everyone we've asked can recall a very important childless person in their lives— whether related or not. Being childfree enables you to redefine yourself so that you can once again be close to children.

And childfree also helps us to redefine the idea of family. For one thing, we can free ourselves from the false notion that two people are not a family, as in the dreaded question, "When are you going to start a family?" Our answer is that we *are* a family, and we hope that something in our tone of voice indicates that we resent the assumption implied in the question that without children we will remain forever incomplete—not a family. We can also free ourselves from the other false notion that children can somehow be *owned,* that they are the *property* of one particular set of parents—and therefore denied to people like us who cannot *produce* them. We are part of the wider family of humankind. Our lives are enriched by the addition of any new life in the world. And the celebrations of rites of passage—births, christenings, brisses, bar mitzvahs, graduations, weddings—are celebrations of the continuation of the life cycle, whether they are our genetic representatives or not. We don't have to "own" members of the younger generation to be delighted by them and vitally interested in their lives. They are *our* hope for a better world, too.

Connie tells of how this insight came to her:

Now that I am childfree, the children of the world are no longer sources of jealous pain, but of joy. They are my stake in the future. This became clear to me one day in the Christmas season. I was listening to Handel's *Messiah* and hearing the chorus sing, "For unto us a Child is born, unto us a Son is given." This is, to me, one of the most beautiful pieces of music on earth, but for years I had been unable to listen to it without crying tears of anger and frustration. But this time I suddenly realized that that particular Child *had* been born to me. I *was* given that Son. I participated in that redemption as much as anyone, fertile or not. It was as if I had been readmitted to the human race.

4. What It Does Not Mean to Live Childfree

After all this positive talk about what we feel is a positive condition, we hate to end on a negative note. But sometimes saying what something *is not* is a way of saying more clearly what it *is.* We also think that a short discussion of what childfree is *not* may be particularly appropriate because our talks to various groups and the letters we have received have convinced us that childfree is a much misunderstood term. Here are some quotes that represent some of those misunderstandings.

"My husband doesn't want to adopt and prefers to live childfree. He does want children if they are our own biologically. I think I would adopt if my husband supported it, but I don't want to push it. So I guess I have to accept a childfree home."

"A few months ago we had to accept the painful fact that we are to remain childfree—a position in life we did not bargain for but none-the-less have to accept."

"I am now stuck living childfree after years of trying and an unsuccessful in vitro attempt. By then it was really too late to try adoption even if I could have convinced my husband to want to, which is unlikely. Also, the attempt totally ruined our sex life. Why yes, I guess I am angry.

"I'm glad to hear your side of the adoption issue aired."

"My husband and I are probably going to be living childfree but not really because we choose to. We are just having to resign ourselves to having no options."

Our understanding of childfree is different.

Childfree does not mean failing or giving up. As we said earlier, childfree means no longer trying to get pregnant, putting that life goal behind you and going on to other things. It means getting off the infertility merry-go-round and walking straight again. But when getting off is seen as failing or giving up, it can't be childfree. "Failing" and "giving up" are terms that imply that the old goal is still of paramount importance, that you are still defining your life by something you don't (and can't) have. Childfree means shifting goals. You let go of a goal that you can't achieve and find other goals that are possible. You are no longer a failure at having children but a success at all the things you can do without children.

Childfree does not mean sad or angry resignation to a childless existence. It's perfectly normal to feel sad or angry (and usually both) about your infertility, but if your sadness and anger continue to dominate the way you feel about your infertility, then you are not really childfree. Childfree comes only when you can put your sadness and anger into perspective. The sadness and anger may never disappear altogether, but you can reconcile yourself to those feelings so that the way you feel about your infertility is dominated by the positive feelings of living without children. Later in the book we will talk about gaining perspective and reconciliation.

Childfree does not mean searching for reasons not to adopt, nor does it mean that you are anti-adoption. And the decision not to adopt does not automatically make you childfree. In fact, we believe that adoption and childfree are separate issues, different ways of resolving an infertility crisis, of becoming no longer infertile. Each one is an affirmation of its own. Childfree is not the negative side of adoption, and adoption is not the negative side of childfree.

Childfree does not mean living without children by decree. So many of the letters we have received told sad stories of no communication between the husband and wife as they go through their infertility crisis. The couple, then, becomes "childfree" because one member says that's the way it will be or, worse, won't even talk about it. (And we are sorry to report that it is the man who usually stops the conversation.) Childfree has to be the result of a lot of communication, often with the help of a counselor. Childfree depends on a mutual sharing that often becomes the basis for a sharing throughout the marriage.

Childfree does not mean coming to the end of your options, having no choices, taking what's left. In fact, our idea of childfree is precisely the opposite. If you've looked ahead at the later chapters in this book, you've seen that choice is a major theme. As strange as it may seem, childfree *must* be the result of a choice.

We will talk a lot more in this book about choice, communication, adoption, sadness and anger, and being a success.

5. Conclusion

The purpose of this chapter was to sketch out our concept of childfree, what it is and what it is not. But we certainly don't want to give the impression that the childfree route to no longer being infertile is quick and easy. Infertility is one of the most traumatic experiences you can endure. It shakes up your life and makes you doubt yourself. It defines you as a failure at one of the most important things you can do with your life. You don't get over something like that by simply declaring yourself childfree.

Becoming childfree takes a lot of work. In the next three chapters we will talk more specifically about what it means to be childfree and the kind of work that it requires.

●

The Transformation
From Childless to Childfree

*I am learning that I am limited as a person only as far as I
allow myself to be; that my happiness does not depend on
having children. I must let go of what I do not have and
concentrate on what I can become.*

—Frankie

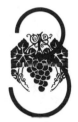

So far we've presented a very
optimistic picture of what it means to
live childfree. It was, for us, the happy
ending to our infertility crisis. After the
silent fears of infertility had turned into
certainty, after all hope of having
children vanished, after the rage and
despair and feelings of inadequacy, our lives are now better than
they have ever been. We don't mean simply bearable or even as
good as before. We mean better. Something good happened in
the change from being infertile to being childfree.

But you may still be doubtful. Perhaps you think that we
are seeing childlessness through rose-colored glasses. Or maybe
you are thinking, it's all fine for them, but what about me? Do
they have evidence that it works that way for anyone else? Of
course, it also occurred to us that we might be just an isolated
case. Perhaps, we joked, the positive changes we found in our
lives were only a shared delusion. But as we talked to people and
read more about it, we discovered that we were not alone. If
childfree is a delusion, then it is a delusion shared by a lot of
people. As it turns out, though, our research has demonstrated
that there was no delusion; our experience of becoming childfree
was a natural result of working through the loss, disappointment,
and stress of a life change.

In this chapter we take a look at this research and the
hope that it offers to people who have suffered the loss of their
fertility. The subject is grief, a subject, we realize, that some
people may find morbid and others just boring. But we hope that
you will bear with us because what we will do here is to offer a
fresh perspective on grief that is both optimistic and exciting. It is

a perspective we wish we had found earlier in our own infertility crisis because it provides the basis for changing infertility into childfree or open to adoption. It explains what it means to stop being infertile.

1. Grief Again: What the Metaphor Misses

If you have read other books on infertility, you have probably come upon an explanation of the infertility crisis as a process of grieving. Most of these explanations are based on Elisabeth Kubler-Ross' studies of terminally ill patients and how they react to their impending deaths. She found that there are five stages that characterize most grief processes: denial and isolation, anger, bargaining, depression, and acceptance. Barbara Eck Menning provides one of the best discussions of the reaction to infertility as a form of grieving.

The idea that infertility sparks a grief reaction has been very helpful to many infertile people. It explains what is happening to us during the infertility crisis and why we feel so bad. We are, in a way, responding to a severe loss that feels like a death. Also, the grief process that Kubler-Ross describes offers hope to those who are grieving, the hope of resolution, the peace that comes with the acceptance of the loss. What we endure when we grieve our loss of fertility—the anger, desolation, rage, fear, depression—is all a part of a process that helps to bring acceptance. What's even more comforting is that it is through these bad feelings that we gain acceptance. Thus, feeling bad about our infertility is okay because it is the way we work through to the resolution of our pain.

When it is seen this way, Kubler-Ross' model of grieving is a valuable means of understanding the infertility crisis. It is an accurate description of the labyrinth that many of us find ourselves in, but it is also a promise that there is a way out of the labyrinth. We can come to peace with our past and with ourselves.

Though it is true that Kubler-Ross' concept of grief has been generally beneficial to understanding the way people respond during an infertility crisis, we found that it is in some ways not appropriate to infertility. For one thing, the Kubler-

Ross model is based specifically on death, which provides a clear focus for grieving. Infertility, however, is what one psychologist calls a deathless death. What makes infertility so painful is that there are so *many* focuses for grief: every trip to the doctor, every pregnant woman we see, every month when the period begins.

An even greater problem we have with the Kubler-Ross model is that it doesn't seem to account for what happened to us when we chose to become childfree. We came to accept our infertility in much the way the model suggests, but the process didn't stop there. Our decision to live childfree took us beyond acceptance to a new affirmation of our lives. We feel that this transformation from accepting our childlessness to becoming childfree left us better off than we were before all the infertility problems began. The process led beyond acceptance to growth, a transformation of the loss into a gain.

This is what we miss in the Kubler-Ross model. In order to understand what being childfree is all about we needed to find a way to account for the transformation to childfree. We found such an account in a book titled *Stress, Loss, and Grief* by the psychologist John Schneider.

2. Stress Reaction: A Different Approach to Grief

Based on his own experience as a clinical psychologist and also the scholarship of other psychologists and counselors, John Schneider offers a model of grieving that seems to be a more appropriate way of describing the reaction to infertility— and what it means to be childfree. He does this by broadening the definition of grief to include reaction to stress caused by life changes. He also shows how grief can take us beyond acceptance to a place where we transform the loss into a gain. It is this view of the grieving process that best accounts for what happens when we become childfree.

Let's begin by looking at the way he broadens the idea of grief to include reaction to stress. Stress is one of those awkward words whose popular meaning is different from the way experts use it. To most of us, stress is something bad, the force in our lives that causes physical and emotional tension. But for psychologists, stress is a neutral term, "any stimulus requiring an organism to adapt to that stimulus." What this means is that stress is what makes us do things; it is something that makes us respond. We all need moderate levels of stress in order to get anything done. Indeed, life without some stress would not be worth living. We may fantasize about getting out of the rat race and retiring to an isolated tropical island, but we don't really want to avoid all stress. Our lives would be boring.

Most of us handle our daily stress well. But there is one kind of stress that usually elicits a grief reaction. Schneider calls this a life-change stress. The reason that grief is the appropriate response to life changes is that almost all life changes, even the "good" ones, bring with them some kind of a loss. And it is perfectly natural—even beneficial—for us human beings to grieve for what we have lost.

At first, this rule that even good life changes involve loss may go against our intuition. What about getting a promotion, celebrating a birthday or anniversary, having children, getting married? What kind of losses are involved in these life-change events? A promotion can also mean the loss of a previous identity at a place of work, no longer being on the same level as many fellow employees. The increased responsibility that comes with a promotion means losing the ability to pass that responsibility to someone else. Birthdays and anniversaries represent the loss of youth and perhaps of opportunities for growth. Getting married can be a severe life change because of the loss of freedom, loss of identification as a single person, and even loss of friends who were an important part of your single life. And having children can bring losses too: further constraints on freedoms, loss of a more easy-going lifestyle, and certainly loss of sleep. Even the holidays that we celebrate can bring with them a feeling of loss. Many people feel depressed at Christmas time, for instance, because of a sense of unfulfilled expectations, of dream Christmases that cannot be found, of special people who are no longer there.

Grieving, even just a little, is a normal response to loss. The problem, says Schneider, is that we tend not to recognize the fact that even "good" life changes bring with them a sense of loss. What happens is that we don't expect the loss and are surprised by feeling sad when by all rights we should be feeling happy. We find ourselves grieving a little and we don't really know why. But it's okay to feel sad, especially when we recognize the loss that comes with life changes and learn to accept those losses as a part of those changes.

This view of grief is also valuable for people who are going through clearly negative life changes such as an infertility crisis. It is valuable because it takes the concept out of the exclusive realm of death and places it in everyday life. For most of us, infertility is a life-change stress. The treatment itself creates changes in our lives: the tests, the calendars, the sex on demand, the scrutiny of all aspects of our lives including the kind of underwear we use. We become different from our friends who have children and fit into the natural life cycle. Our lives seem to have one all-encompassing focus, which makes jobs, hobbies, friends—all the things we used to define ourselves by—secondary. In fact, we begin to see ourselves as failures at the most important aspect of our lives, which has a way of poisoning with failure other aspects as well.

All these changes add up to a lot of stress and feelings of loss, and grief is the way we react to both. But what's important here is that it is not only the metaphoric death of a child (though in some instances, such as in the case of a miscarriage, this is no longer metaphoric) or of the dreams of having a child; rather, it is also the loss that is associated with the stress of a severe life change. What makes us feel bad is not so much the loss of a child as it is the loss of a self identity, the control of our bodies and of our destinies. Grief is how we react to that loss. We feel bad. We hurt. We get depressed and angry. And that's okay because grief is a natural response to the loss that comes with a life change.

To us, this view of grief makes more sense as a way of understanding infertility than the view of grief as a reaction to death. Infertility brought about major changes in our lives, changes that added up to a lot of loss. Sure we felt bad, but there was a good reason for it: our grief was a natural response to the overwhelming stress of infertility. Because it freed us from associations with death, this broader concept of the source of grief provided us with a more helpful understanding of why infertility hurt so much.

Schneider's Three "Tasks" of Grieving

Task 1   **Limiting the Awareness of the Loss**
                Two Denial Strategies
                    1. Letting Go
                    2. Holding On

Task 2   **Gaining Some Perspective on the Loss**
                    1. Becoming aware of the loss and
                       mourning it
                    2. Coming to accept the loss

Task 3   **Finding the Opportunity for Gain in the Loss**
                    1. Reformulation: Redefining the loss
                    2. Transformation: Affirming the loss,
                       turning it into gain

Figure One   The initial knowledge of a loss usually leads to an
                attempt to limit the awareness of it so that it
                doesn't hurt quite so much. Soon, though, most
                people are able to face the loss and mourn it,
                eventually coming to accept it. However, some
                people will find that the hurt is too great and will
                temporarily return to the previous phase of denial.
                Acceptance typically comes with time, but
                it's possible to go beyond acceptance to a
                transformation of the loss into gain. This step
                usually takes some work on the part of the griever.
                For us, transformation describes the state in
                which the loss of fertility is turned into the gain of
                living childfree or being open to adoption.

3. Transformation

This broader view of grieving helps us to see grief in a more realistic—and applicable—way. But even more important for this book is Schneider's description of the stages of grief, a model that goes beyond Kubler-Ross' acceptance and in doing so provides the basis for understanding what it means to be childfree. We have seen that "good" life changes bring with them the potential for loss. The good news, psychologists tell us, is that the reverse is also true: a loss also possesses the potential for gain. Even though the focus of "bad" life changes is on loss, we should be aware that we have the ability to turn that loss into something positive.

This is a very hopeful view of grief. Certainly, loss is an inevitable part of living, but the possibility that we can turn the pain of loss into something good helps us to see loss in a new light. Instead of something to avoid or ignore, loss can be a way for us to grow personally and as a couple, a clear statement of the power of human beings not only to adapt but to triumph.

Schneider does a good job of helping us to see how the grief process can lead to growth. He describes what he calls the three tasks or phases of grieving. The first two of these tasks are in many ways similar to the stages in the Kubler-Ross model, but the last goes beyond that model and provides the key to no longer being infertile.

During the first phase, the main task of the person who is suffering a loss is to limit the awareness of the loss. This phase must begin, of course, with an initial awareness of the loss or impending loss, an awareness that is often accompanied by a mental and, depending on the severity of the loss, perhaps even physical shock. The natural reaction to a stress that causes a major disruption of normal life is to try to control the situation by limiting awareness of the loss. People in this situation usually fall back on the defensive strategies of holding on or letting go, both of which serve as means of denial.

Holding on is a strategy by which people attempt to cope with a loss either by ignoring it or by trying to direct their energies in another direction. They try to hold on to the status quo in order to limit the change in their lives, thus avoiding the impact of the loss. Letting go, the other denial mechanism, is a strategy through which people try to cope with their loss by minimizing that loss as much as possible. They convince themselves that what they have lost is not important anyway. They detach themselves from it or dwell on its negative aspects. This is a perfectly natural way of reacting so that the experience of loss will be less overpowering.

Both holding on and letting go are normal responses to the pain of a loss or a potential loss. It hurts and we want to limit the hurt. However, when people rely too much on these coping mechanisms, they become stagnated in this phase, unable to take their grief any further. The problem with this is that while we are holding on or letting go, grief cannot run its beneficial course. You can't grieve as long as you deny that there is a loss.

Of the many stories we have heard from infertile couples, we have found that it is usually the husband who gets stuck in the denial phase. Esther wrote to us without her husband knowing it. She said, "He apparently, doesn't have the same need to share these intolerable feelings as I do. Perhaps that is because the problem is mine. Who knows? Perhaps he will divorce me some day and marry a woman who *can* bear him children." Later she confided, "I'm so tired of discussing anything that has to do with 'our' problem that I wonder if I should become an ostrich, like my husband, and ignore it—only I can't."

Esther's ironic description of "our" problem captures the essence of her pain. Her husband's holding-on strategy is a way of denying that their infertility is a problem, or at least *his* problem. The trouble is that his denial is causing her to suffer alone. She can't ignore the hurt, but because her husband won't allow her to talk about it, she also cannot work through the hurt toward acceptance of the loss. There is no way that she can heal all by herself because she feels responsible and also fears that he will leave her. It's a painful story, but it illustrates so well the fact that for an infertile couple, grieving must be a mutual act. They must allow for real communication, even if it does hurt, to eventually get out of the denial phase.

In the second phase of grief, Schneider describes the task of the griever as gaining some perspective on the loss and thus coming to accept it. Because it is perfectly natural to limit pain, it is also perfectly natural to limit the awareness of the loss. But in most people, there comes a time when all attempts at denial have been exhausted and they must face the reality of their loss. Facing loss is what we call mourning. People feel lonely, isolated, helpless, and empty. Often these feelings are episodic: there are periods when they seem to forget the loss, but there are also periods when awareness comes flooding back and brings with it renewed feelings of sadness and depression.

The important message, though, is that it's okay to mourn, to feel the despair, hopelessness, and even depression that comes with the loss. It's okay because psychologists tell us that it is through this awareness of loss that we come to accept it, to make peace with it. The mourning may be rather short, such as when your favorite basketball team loses in the NCAA tournament, or it may be long, as with the death of a child or spouse. However long it is, though, most people eventually find that they have come to accept the loss.

This acceptance is usually passive, beginning with a feeling of resignation in the face of the inevitable. It is a matter of gaining some perspective on the loss, the ability to see both the positive and the negative aspects of it and the acceptance of what responsibility there may be, your own and others'. Another characteristic of this acceptance is forgiveness, forgiving yourself and others. The interesting thing about this acceptance and the healing that comes with it is that it is usually not something that can be willed and it does not occur dramatically. People often just realize that in time they feel better. Their tension is gone, they have more energy available to them, and they find a fresh sense of freedom and hope for themselves.

An illustration of this acceptance is provided by Sonya Sochor and her husband, who realized that they had accepted their childlessness when they were in the market for a new house.

> When we began to house hunt in Muncie, the realtor showed us numerous houses similar to the very traditional family-type house that we had in Columbus (large family room, three bedrooms, fenced-in backyard). We seemed to find fault with every one of them, and none of them really felt "like home" when we walked in. The one that felt "like

home" and the one that we finally did choose, is more a couple's house than a family's house. There is no family room, the backyard enters onto a nicely carpeted great room, not at all practical for sandboxes and wading pools. As well, there is no empty room here, as in Columbus, waiting to be turned into a nursery.

Acceptance marked the end of their mourning.

It is to the point of acceptance that Kubler-Ross' model takes us. But many researchers (including Kubler-Ross in her later work, *Death: The Final Stage of Growth*) have found that there is an additional potential for taking the grief process beyond acceptance. Schneider finds that this often occurs in two stages. The first stage is the reformulation of the loss, which is an outgrowth of acceptance. Reformulation means redefining the loss. It is taking the understanding and the energy that one finds in acceptance and shifting perspectives "from focusing on limits to focusing on potential; from coping to growth; and from problems to challenges." Reformulation means gaining an entirely new attitude toward the loss and a renewed strength for carrying on. The individual or couple finds in their acceptance of loss the opportunity for personal gain and with it the understanding that we can't have everything we want.

The second stage in this last phase of grieving is the transformation of loss into gain. Whereas most of the grief process up to this point has been focused inward, the transformation stage tends to be focused outward, moving the griever into the wider realm of humanity. Schneider describes it this way: "Transforming loss involves the person placing the loss in a context of growth, life cycles and the view that grief is a unifying rather than an alienating human experience."

Transformation is the key to this hopeful view of grief. The second phase of grieving led to an acceptance of the loss, a natural result of facing the loss and mourning it. You eventually find that you have come to accept it. But it is in the final phase of grief that acceptance may be transformed into affirmation. You can affirm the loss, you can embrace it, because of the gain that it now brings. Instead of a source of pain, the loss becomes an opportunity for growth.

At first, this may seem like a strange and esoteric way of looking at grief, but when you get used to it, it is startlingly sensible. Basically, it is a process of changing perception, from a narrow focus on the individual griever to a broader focus that encompasses all humanity. The limited awareness phase is a time of negative perception in which the task is *not* to know. The second phase is characterized by a growth in perception, a concentration on the loss and how it makes the griever feel— angry, sad, depressed. In learning to accept the loss, the focus is still very much on the individual and perhaps a small group of related others—accepting responsibility, forgiving, saying goodbye. Reformulation begins to expand the griever's perceptions from the past to the future and enhances the opportunities for personal growth.

The process of changing perspective concludes in transormation, which takes the griever beyond the individuality of the loss to a perception that embraces the wider human experience in which, as Schneider says, "people are connected to all things by means of love, commitments, and cycles of continuity with past, present, and future." Instead of seeing the loss in terms of the disruption of lives, we come to see it as connecting us to the larger forces of life. The loss, then, becomes a source for growth and wider understanding. Indeed, the loss is turned into a gain as the energy we had invested in the old attachment is freed to be used in other ways. Transformation means emerging from grief as a fuller, richer, growing person. It is the process of taking a significant loss and turning it into a significant gain. This transformation of the loss of fertility into the gain that can come with being childfree is described by Anne I. Smith:

> The childfree decision is a very difficult one to make, but it can be a very rewarding decision for the infertile couple. It can release you to a new exciting and rewarding life. My husband, Doug, and I have come to accept our situation. We've grieved through the loss of our dream and have made the decision to be childfree. I now have an inner peace and outer

excitement about life that I haven't had in eight years. Life will go on with meaning and purpose. I now have control over my life. The door has been closed on eight years of unhappiness, and a new door is opening to a happy and rewarding life because of this decision.

4. How All of This Helps Us to Understand Childfree

Schneider's model of grief is very useful in helping people understand how they react to any loss. For us, though, it has some very important implications for the specific loss of fertility.

First, it helps us to understand why infertility affects us the way it does. Infertility is a major, and for some of us catastrophic, life change. And like any other life change, the loss of our fertility is stressful, a disruption of our lives. Grief is the way that human beings deal with stress and loss. And, generally speaking, the more disruptive the stress and the more we value what we have lost, the more intense our grief reaction will be. Stress and loss—these are a good ways of describing an infertility crisis. And, naturally, we grieve. This model broadens the grief process to include reactions to loss other than death—such as the loss of fertility.

The second insight we can draw from this model relates more specifically to what this book is all about—how to stop being infertile. Schneider's transformation of loss into gain is what we mean when we talk about the transformation from childless into childfree. Childlessness belongs to the second phase of the model, a dwelling on the loss and an eventual acceptance of the loss. But even in acceptance, the emphasis is still on being child*less*. It is an acceptance of the *loss*. In the transformation phase of the model, the emphasis shifts from acceptance to affirmation. Affirmation means embracing your childlessness as a positive, freeing thing. It is through this affirmation that you become childfree. It means seeing childlessness not as a punishment or a cruel trick of fate but as an opportunity for growth. It means finding that life is good again and taking advantage of not having children to make it even better.

We realize that for many of you these words may seem empty and perhaps even painful in contrast to the way you are feeling now. If so, we are sorry. But what we hope is that you can also see the hopefulness that is inherent in this model. There is the possibility for a happy ending to your infertility story. One happy ending could be having a biological child. Another could be adopting a child. Or you may find your happy ending in choosing to live childfree. The grief model we have described offers the possibility that childfree living can be a happy ending too.

The third lesson this model offers is that grieving one loss is, in many ways, the same as grieving another loss. Schneider demonstrates the significance of that similarity by showing that the way we grieve one loss influences the way we grieve other losses. For some of us, infertility is the greatest loss that we have faced. The experts tell us, however, that the way we handle the loss of our fertility is an indication of how we will handle the other losses that will surely occur in our lives. Grief is, to a large degree, a learned behavior. If we can seize the possibilities for growth in this crisis, there is every indication that we will do the same for other crises we will face. Dealing successfully with this loss gives us the hope of greater strength and understanding in dealing with other losses. If we can learn how to see the potential for gain in all loss, we will have learned one of the greatest lessons of living.

5. Conclusion

Schneider's discussion of stress, loss, and grief was a revelation to us. We had witnessed our own reaction to infertility, we had read or heard about others', but we had no idea what was really going on or even if the state we were calling childfree actually existed. How could we talk about living childfree if all we could rely on was anecdotal evidence? All we could do was what we have done in the first two chapters—provide a few definitions and stories and hope that something clicked with our readers.

Schneider's model of grief changed all that. It proved to us that childfree was not just a word a few people dreamed up to make themselves feel better. Childfree really signified something. And it's not something mysterious and elusive; on the contrary, it is a normal step in a reaction to the loss of fertility, the transformation from loss to gain. What's especially important in this is that as a transformation, childfree is a part of a larger grief process. Childfree is not something special and therefore suspect. It is the potential for gain that comes with any significant loss.

The potential for gain in loss has valuable implications for us not just as infertile people but as human beings. The problem is that not everyone achieves this potential. Most people learn to accept their losses, even great losses, because acceptance usually comes in time. It is a natural result of mourning. But the transformation from loss to gain is more rare. The reason is that transformation doesn't just happen; it requires a lot of work, a lot of time, a lot of communication, and often it requires the help of a counselor. In the next two chapters we will look at some of the work that goes into achieving the transformation from loss to gain.

Loss is an inevitable part of life. But that doesn't mean that life is meaningless suffering. Schneider's model of grief helps us to see the true potential of loss—that instead of simply enduring, we can prevail.

●

WOMEN'S COLLEGE HOSPITAL
WOMEN'S HEALTH CENTRE
THE RESOURCE CENTRE

The Power of Choice: Making Life Decisions

Everything, at least every important thing that happens to us, is a snippet in our continued story, the life story we are writing with our choices.
—Lewis B. Smedes

As we saw in the last chapter, childfree may be defined as the final stage in the grief process, a rebirth that transforms acceptance into affirmation. The next logical question is how can you achieve this transformation? Unfortunately, there is no magic formula or 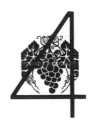 series of steps to follow. But if we had to come up with one basic necessity for transforming childless into childfree, it would be choice; you have to choose childfree in order to live childfree.

There are, of course, many choices that infertile couples must make: whether or not and when to seek medical help, what doctor to go to, what kind of treatments to take, when to stop treatments, whether or not to adopt, and others. As we go through our infertility workups, the decisions get more and more difficult. Treatment becomes more complicated and more risky. Stopping treatment is a radical step that may feel like giving up. Deciding to adopt and what method of adoption to use has implications for how we spend the rest of our lives.

In this chapter, we will discuss what it means to choose to live childfree. We may not be able to offer easy guidelines for becoming childfree, but we can offer you the hope that it can be done and give you some suggestions for making such life choices. These suggestions come chiefly from Dr. Theodore Rubin's book, *Overcoming Indecisiveness.* Dr. Rubin is a psychiatrist whose work on making decisions meshes very well with John Schneider's model of grief that we talked about in the last chapter. Basically the two theories work togther this way: *the life stress that comes from loss may be transformed into gain through the process of making a life decision.*

1. Thinking about Ending Your Infertility

As we said, there are many decisions that couples have to make during their infertility workup. There are three related choices, however, that most infertile couples tend to ignore until late in the infertility journey: stopping treatment, adopting, and living childfree. The reason these choices are ignored is that infertile couples hope that they won't have to make such decisions. And, in fact, the chances are good that they won't. But instead of ignoring these choices, we think that it's important to anticipate them, to understand their implications and the way they relate to each other.

Our friends Janice and Carl Cowen have spoken very perceptively about the decision to stop treatment. They make several important points. First, everybody stops treatment at some time. Infertility, by its nature, is limited. Couples may stop treatment because they have a child or because the risks and effectiveness of continued treatment are not worth it. Second, it's okay to stop treatment without making a child. Stopping treatment is not giving up; it's not failure. It's a very reasonable decision that couples make when the risks and expense outweigh the possible benefits. A third point is that the decision to stop treatment should be the result of active decision making. Such a decision cannot be made by default, simply giving up. Instead, it should be seen as a choice that both members of the couple must share, a mutual act that is based on open, trusting communication.

It's also important to see adoption as a choice, not just the next logical step after stopping treatment. Adoption is not for everybody. It requires a commitment that can come only from making a serious, conscious decision. The decision to adopt should indicate that the couple *wants* to adopt and is not adopting simply because nothing else has worked. The decision to adopt should also be a sign that the couple has embraced their own childlessness and is willing to see their adopted child not as a substitute for what they can't otherwise have but as a person whom they can accept on his or her own terms. This has to be the result of a choice.

Each of these decisions has this feature in common— each one is a life choice. They are also related because they come at the end of the infertility process. But it's important also to see them as separate. The decision to stop treatment is not the same as to adopt or to live childfree. And the decision *not* to adopt is not the same as the decision to live childfree, which, we think, must be a positive one, not simply the decision *not* to do something else.

It's tempting to try to put these choices in some order that would indicate a clear process for ending the infertility workup. Unfortunately, though, it's not that easy. The Cowens suggest that making the decision to stop treatment may often be the catalyst for making decisions about what alternatives to follow. But they point out that it is not a matter of putting off consideration of alternatives until after deciding to stop treatment: "Although it might look appealing to make the decision to stop and then consider what you will do instead, you will find that you need to consider what the alternatives are as you are considering whether to stop." This is what we did. We had found out about alternatives to having biological children long before we decided to stop our infertility workup. But it was the decision to stop that made us start considering the alternatives seriously.

There may be no set order for considering these life decisions, but we can recommend one thing that may make the decisions easier: think about them ahead of time. You will stop treatment at some point, and the chances are good that it will be because you will get pregnant. But whether you like it or not, it's a good idea at least to consider the possibility that you might not be able to have a biological child.

You may want to anticipate the decision to stop treatment by beginning to talk about the limits to risk and expense and emotional damage that you want to place on the treatment. It's your decision. You may also want to anticipate what alternatives you will want to follow after stopping treatment. Perhaps some form of adoption. You will want to start talking about whether adoption is for you, find out how it is done, talk to others who have adopted. Perhaps childfree. You need to investigate that alternative, too. Find out what it means to be childfree, find some childfree couples who can serve as role models, try it on and see if it fits *you*.

The other alternative is making no decision at all, a condition that we call drifting. Though we have no hard evidence to support it, our experience tells us that most infertile couples who don't have children, genetic or adopted, end up as drifters. These are people who don't *decide* to stop treatment; they just don't bother to go to the doctor any more. They don't *decide* not to adopt, they just never get around to it, or, more likely, one of them will object to adoption and just leave it that way. And they don't *decide* to live childfree; *they remain childless.*

The point is that it's important, even early in the infertility workup and treatment, to think about the future because there is life after infertility—and you can make it a good life. It's necessary to anticipate the future because life decisions are so much easier to make when they are grounded in some forethought. It's important to talk about these possibilities. It's also important to see these decisions in a positive light, not as a failure to achieve a goal or as giving up hope. It is by making life decisions that we can stop being infertilie.

2. The Paradox of Choice

In our conversations with infertile people, we've discovered that the paradoxical nature of choosing to live childfree is difficult to understand. One woman captured the confusion this way: "When you say you chose to *affirm* the decision to live childfree, I'm not sure what you mean. After all, you weren't given the choice at all. You were unable to conceive." How can you *choose* what you already have and don't want? This is a paradox.

But a paradox is an apparent contradiction that is nevertheless true. The emphasis in that sentence is obviously on *apparent.* What we will try to do here is explain in what way the paradox of choosing childfree is actually true.

John Schneider's model of grief addresses this issue of choice. He says that the first two tasks of grief—limiting awareness and acceptance—both imply a fatalistic or deterministic view of life. This means that we must resign ourselves to our fate, whatever it is, because we have little or no control over our lives. But he also says that the transformation to affirmation "implies the potential for free will or at least the freedom to view life as containing choices. It assumes that people are capable of choosing, even in the face of overwhelming loss or evidence of impending death, and that they can choose not only to live but to what extent."

This is a very hopeful view of life—that human beings, even in the face of great loss, can reassert control over their lives and find meaning and purpose once again. And, as Schneider suggests, this depends on seeing our lives as containing choices. It is only through choice that we can exert the control over our lives that leads to the transformation from loss to gain.

Schneider provides another way of understanding how choice works in the grief process. He describes acceptance as something that comes to most people quite naturally. Once they allow themselves to feel the pain of the loss, time eventually brings its healing acceptance of the loss. Affirmation is different, though. It demands active participation in the grief process—the work involved in making a choice. Life decisions do not come easily or casually; they demand that we not only take the time and effort to go through a decision-making process but also invest ourselves fully in the decision we make. It is this active participation that distinguishes acceptance from affirmation.

We would also like to contradict the old adage that not to decide is to decide. The implication is that simply drifting along in a situation could be interpreted as a choice to remain in that situation. Dr. Rubin says that this is not true: not to decide is to abdicate responsibility, which can lead to feelings of paralysis and failure. People who are abdicators lose the opportunity to give direction to their lives. The value of making life decisions, then, is that you own more of yourself. The fact is that people who make life decisions have greater control over their lives than people who don't. The decisions we make actually define us, a collective statement of who we are. But if we avoid making decisions we abdicate responsibility for ourselves and remain, in a way, undefined.

So choice plays a crucial role in the transformation from childless to childfree. It is a way of regaining control over our lives, of affirming who we are. When we look at choice in this light, the contradiction of the paradox begins to disappear. It would be a *real* contradiction to say that you could choose to be childless when you couldn't have children. To be child*free*, though, *demands* a choice. The transformation from acceptance of childlessness to childfree occurs through the process of making a life decision. It is not simply resigning yourself to your fate. It is not the stoic acceptance of what you can't change. No, it is the act of making a decision to create a positive change.

And what does it mean to choose to live childfree? It means embracing your childlessness as a positive state, as an opportunity for growth, as a path to greater achievement and happiness. It means no longer defining yourself as infertile, no longer seeing yourself in terms of what you don't have. It means changing failure into success, negative into positive. It means reclaiming the energy that allows you to be yourself again.

Now, let's look at Rubin's three tasks for making a life decision.

3. Task Number One: Identifying and Removing Decision Blockers

If, as Dr. Rubin says, decisions are the way we gain control over our lives, why is it that many people have so much difficulty making decisions? There are several possible answers to that question. One is that claiming control over our lives also means taking responsibility for our lives. Often, it's easier to see ourselves as tossed about on the sea of fate, out of control but also not responsible. It's easy to blame others or fate or God, but it takes a lot of maturity to shoulder your own responsibility.

Another reason is that it takes a lot of work to make life decisions and demands risk as well. Making life decisions, particularly decisions that also affect others, requires communication—extensive communication— and communication requires the ability to open yourself up so that you can express your own feelings and understand another person's feelings. It's certainly easier to ignore a life stress or to sit idly by while someone else does all the work. It is through decision making, though, that we take responsibility for our lives.

These reasons are certainly too broad and too personal for us to deal with here. But Dr. Rubin does outline other difficulties with making life decisions that we can talk about. He calls them decision blockers, obstacles that tend to get in our way

Rubin's Three "Tasks" for Making Life Decisions

Task 1   **Identifying and Overcoming Decision Blockers**
1. Losing touch with feelings
2. Resignation
3. Depression
4. Dom Perignon Syndrome
5. Procrastination
6. The "Coulda, Woulda, Shoulda" Syndrome
7. Option blindness

Task 2   **Establishing a Foundation for Decision Making: Your Priorities**

Task 3   **Committing Yourself to Your Decision**
1. Registering your decision
2. Investing yourself in your decision

Figure Two   These three "tasks" will guide you in making the life decisions associated with infertility. First, you look for obstacles to decision making and deal with them. Second, you redefine yourself by studying your priorities, the keys to your values. Finally, you follow through on your decision, committing yourself to living by it.

and keep us from making decisions. It's necessary, if we are going to make a life decision, to recognize and remove the obstacles that may be in the way. Here are some of Rubin's decision blockers that infertile couples may find especially applicable.

The first blocker is the result of losing touch with feelings. This is a kind of alienation that often comes from living with pain. Such a reaction is natural, of course. If something is painful, your first response is to distance yourself from it. You simply don't allow yourself to feel, a denial that the pain exists. There are two problems associated with this kind of decision blocker. One is that pain often serves as the stimulus that makes us decide something. If we deny the pain, then we lose the drive to make the decision that allows us to get out of the situation. The other problem is that we can't make a decision if we cut ourselves off from our feelings. The trouble with distancing ourselves from pain is that we tend to distance ourselves from everything else. We lose all our feelings. Making a decision demands that we open ourselves up to our feelings. But this is worth it because it is by making a decision that we can begin to take the pain away.

The second blocker is a different kind of reaction to pain—resignation. People who resign themselves to a bad situation are actually trying to avoid conflict and choice. They see choice as something bad, tearing them apart. Resignation is often the result of a fear of change, an overwhelming desire to maintain the status quo. It is characterized by detachment; it keeps us from knowing ourselves. Resignation is another way of hiding from a bad situation. But the main problem is that resignation stymies all motivation for making a change.

Another decision blocker is depression. When you're depressed, you feel stuck, constantly tired, hopeless, sad, and anxious. You lose your appetite and the ability to feel joy and pleasure. You feel bored, guilty, preoccupied with loss. It is impossible to get any perspective on a situation when you are depressed. Making a decision is a statement of hope and of faith in the future. Depression does not allow for such hope and faith.

If these three decision blockers sound familiar it's because you recognize them from Schneider's model of grief. Losing touch with feelings is the same as the denial stage of letting go. Resignation, the avoidance of change by maintaining the status quo, corresponds to the other denial stage of holding on. And clearly the depression is from the mourning phase of the model. All these are, of course, legitimate and appropriate reactions to loss. Loss is painful, so we try to hide from the pain. And when we begin to feel the pain of the loss, we feel depressed.

The problem is that it's possible to get stuck in one of these stages. Then, making a decision becomes very difficult. The reason for this is quite simple: before you can embrace the decision to stop treatment, to adopt, or to live childfree, you need to accept the loss of your biological child. You can't effectively make these life decisions without that acceptance, which, as Schneider shows, is a prerequisite to transformation. If you feel like you or your spouse is stuck in the denial or the depression stage, we recommend that you both get some counseling. For some people, especially those who are deep in denial, this may be difficult. A gentle push from a loved one, however, might be just the touch it would take to get help.

But even if you have come to the point of accepting your loss and have the impetus to make a decision, there are other blockers that can get in your way.

One of these blockers is what Rubin calls the Dom Perignon Syndrome, after the premium-grade champagne. This syndrome comes in two different, shall we say, "vintages." One is the demand that everything that you do be correct. We all know perfectionists, but this particular kind has a problem making decisions because he or she fears that the decision might be wrong. This leads to decision paralysis. One thing that we have learned is that in most cases there are no absolute right or wrong decisions, which is a freeing concept for people afflicted with this kind of paralysis. More on this later.

The other "vintage" is the desire to have it all. This creates another kind of decision paralysis because every decision to do one thing is inevitably a decision *not* to do another. It's true that you can't eat you cake and have it too; for every door you open you leave many more forever closed. Part of choosing to live childfree is choosing to live without children. There's no way to get around that. But it is important to see not only that there is within every loss the potential for gain but also that in every gain there is an inevitable loss. The inability to accept that loss, even when the gain is clear, keeps some people from making any decision.

Another of Dr. Rubin's blockers that seems particularly appropriate to infertile couples is the persistent belief that something better will come along or that something will happen to erase the whole problem. This is a particularly insidious form of procrastination, a way of avoiding having to make a decision. For infertile couples, this kind of block is best expressed in the hope for a medical miracle, which keeps couples trying new treatments no matter how little chance for success or how risky, physically and emotionally. People who suffer from this syndrome refuse to consider stopping treatment, always believing that just around the corner is a treatment that will work. An even more destructive characteristic of this kind of blocker is the tendency for couples to keep hoping and trying to get pregnant just in case the doctors were wrong, seeking a miracle birth by "relaxing" or a special douche or some other "cure." This kind of hope against all odds may be the material for great stories, but it can also lead to a monthly cycle of hope and despair that can paralyze your life.

Infertile couples, like aging athletes, should know when it is time to bow out gracefully. Growing old is not a crime and neither is putting your infertility behind you. Stopping treatment and getting off the infertility roller coaster is not an admission of failure. In fact, we would say that the reverse is true: you define yourselves as failures when you continue treatment beyond any reasonable expectation or persist in the monthly cycle of hope and despair long after that hope becomes a liability. Success, on the other hand, is knowing when to stop trying to get pregnant; it can free your energy to make a decision and to do something positive with your life.

Rubin describes another decision blocker that may sound familiar to some infertile couples—the "coulda, woulda, shoulda" blocker. This is a paralysis that is founded on guilt, blaming yourself or others for sins (imaginary or not) of omission or comission. Guilt over waiting too long to try to get pregnant. Guilt for having had an abortion. Guilt for not successfully completing a particular treatment that made you sick. Guilt for not wanting a child badly enough. Unfortunately for infertile couples, there seems to be more than enough guilt to go around (again, real or imaginary). Perhaps the worst kind is the guilt that one member of the couple, the one who is "responsible" for the infertility, takes on as a means of contrition. Such contrition requires him or her always to be a little depressed and willing to do anything it takes to get pregnant, no matter what.

Until you can free yourself from the quicksand of guilt, you cannot make a life decision. Clearly what is needed is an act of forgiveness. But often the hardest person to forgive is yourself. We think that a major part of accepting the loss of your fertility is to forgive yourself, to forgive your spouse, and to forgive anyone else who appears blameworthy. Not only does real forgiveness feel good, but it also frees up your energies for more productive means of coping with infertility. But if you are having some difficulty pulling yourself out of the quicksand, you will find that a counselor can help.

The last of Rubin's decision blockers we want to talk about is option blindness, a blocker that gets right to the heart of why many people don't make decisions. Making a decision depends on knowing that there are options, because without options there is no decision to make. Sometimes the most difficult part of making a decision is realizing that a choice is possible. The Cowens have helped us to see that stopping treatment is an option. It's something you can choose. You can also choose to get off the destructive cycle of hope and despair by using birth control again. But the option blindness that most infertile people suffer from concerns living childfree. Earlier in this chapter we mentioned the woman who didn't understand what we meant by *choosing* childfree. "After all," she said, "you weren't given the choice at all. You were unable to conceive."

This confusion is typical of the option blindness that plagues the childfree decision. It is essential to understand first that you *can* choose to live childfree. It is an option, an alternative to living child*less*. But it is also essential to understand that to live childfree demands a choice. It is only through choice that you can be childfree because *it is the act of choosing that gives you control over your life.*

If you want to make a life decision, a good way to begin is to survey the possible decision blockers that might inhibit your ability to make that decision. We have listed here seven decision blockers that seem especially appropriate to people who are trying to make decisions related to their infertility. We have also tried to point out directions you may take toward overcoming these blockers. But if you find that you have trouble doing this on your own, you may want to see a counselor. (We've said this before and we'll say it again.) A counselor can help you make life decisions.

4. Task Number Two: Establishing a Foundation for Decision Making

Freeing yourself from decision blockers puts you in the position to make a life decision. But even at that point you need to have a basis for making a decision. Dr. Rubin says that we make life decisions based on our priorities. Thinking about the priorities for our lives is really a matter of looking at our values, because what we value determines what our priorities are. This is an important connection to make. Rubin points out that we *are* our priorities; we are defined by what we value. You might recall also that a key part of transformation in Schneider's model was redefinition. Looking at our priorities, then, is how we begin to redefine ourselves, which gives us a basis for making a choice.

For infertile couples, this issue of priorities is doubly important because one of the effects of infertility is that our priorities can become skewed, twisted all out of proportion. Infertility tends to give us tunnel vision. Some of us become obsessed; we have one great goal that guides our lives: getting pregnant. The pursuit of this one great goal changes everything. It is *the* priority in our lives, outweighing all the others. If it is true that our priorities define us, then we infertile couples become defined by our quest for fertility, able to see little else of value in our lives, often forsaking or altering what we had previously held valuable.

To make a decision, though, it is necessary to get back in touch with other priorities. Infertility can be a blindfold. It can keep us from seeing our lives from a broader perspective because having a baby overshadows all other priorities. To make a life decision about infertility, we must begin to redefine ourselves as whole people once again, to recognize that there are other priorities in our lives besides having children.

One way of getting in touch with your priorities is to make a list of the things that you think are important in your life. You might even try to rank your top ten priorities. As an aid to making such a list, Rubin offers what he calls the common priorities, the typical things that people call their priorities. His list includes these priorities (and a few we've added):

Health	Religion
Sex	Physical Activity
Work	Intellectual Activity
Money	Creative Activity
Sociability	Appearance
Prestige, Power, and Recognition	Pleasure
	Romance
Education	Making the World a Better Place
Property or Material Things	
Excitement, Stimulation and Variety	Freedom from Stress
	Physical Comfort and Convenience
Contributing to the Welfare of Others	Security
Quality of Life	

Making a list of your priorities can help in two ways. First, it helps you redefine yourself as a full human being once again by getting you to identify the other things in life, besides having a baby, that define you. Second, it helps you make the specific life decisions related to infertility. Stopping treatment, for instance. It's important to get in touch with your priorities in order to determine the point where the value of continuing to apply medical treatment begins to be outweighed by other values. Of course your health is important. But how important is it? What is the point at which you are no longer willing to risk your health to get a baby? It's helpful to keep in mind the balance between infertility treatment and risk to health so that you can make the decision to stop treatment when you get to the point that the risk is too great.

Other priorities are also relevant in the decision to stop

treatment. Sex, romance, freedom from stress, physical comfort and convenience—all of these and others may be threatened at some point by continuing medical treatment. There comes a time for many of us when we must make that decision. It's vital for us to take off our blindfolds and really look at what we want out of our lives. Sometimes, wanting a child of our genetic structure starts to threaten the other things that we desire, things that make our lives worth living.

Your list of priorities can also be used as a basis for making the decision to live childfree. It encourages you to look at the other things in your life that are important and to see how they stack up against having children. Having children, of course, is a wonderful thing, but it's still important to keep it in perspective. There are other things that can make our lives rich and fulfilling. Indeed, it is true that having children may even reduce the opportunity for living out some of our priorities. For some people, work may be important enough for them to realize that having children will be a sacrifice. Money, prestige, power and recognition, education, intellectual and creative activity, appearance, excitement, stimulation, and variety (such as travel), quality of life—all these and many other priorities as well may help you to see the possibilities of living childfree. This renewed sense of perspective may reaffirm your desire to have children by some other method, or it may help you to see that your life can be good without children.

For example, Carol and Robert Vercollone reported that quality of life was a priority that led them to choose to live childfree. Carol writes: "One reason I love my childfree life style is that a peaceful home is important to me. Rob and I are both intensely involved with people in our careers, and we enjoy that. But we also enjoy coming home to either alone time or time to focus on just each other."

When you think about it, this act of looking at the positive side of not having children is what the transformation from childless to childfree is all about. Remember the principle about loss that we talked about in the previous chapter: for every loss there is the potential for gain. What childfree means to us is finding the gain that comes with the loss of fertility, seeing within the negative the possibility for something positive.

One way of doing this is to look at the values that guide

your life to see what of these can be enhanced by not having children. If you find such values, then you have the foundation for living childfree.

But what if you can't find alternative values to build a new life on? What if you are someone who has defined yourself in terms of having children and can't seem to see your life in any other way? And what if you prefer not to adopt? We think that you can still choose to live childfree. In the next chapter we will discuss the various needs that drive us to have children and how to meet those needs in other ways.

5. The Third Task: Committing Yourself to Your Decision

Dr. Rubin says that the decision itself usually doesn't come like a lightening bolt. What typically happens is that after a lot of thinking and talking about the decision, we simply realize that we have made a choice. It feels right. There is a sense of things falling into place, of new-found satisfaction. We feel good about committing ourselves to something that feels right. Indeed, if a decision feels forced or contrived—not quite right for us— then it is probably not a real decision. But if we feel good about it and it feels right for us, then it is a real decision, one we can not only live with but also live by.

This is the way it happened to us. There was no identifiable eureka moment. After all the searching and talking, childfree just felt right. It was the alternative we wanted to follow because it was right for us. It set us on a positive course and gave us a way to get on with the rest of our lives. It fit us.

But even when you realize that you have made a decision, it's important to commit yourself to it, to make it your own. One way of doing this is to "register" the decision, to make it "official." Merle Bombardieri suggests that you do something special to mark your decision to be childfree (or to stop treatment or to adopt). You might go out to dinner to toast the end of your infertility.

Another way of registering your decision is to tell other people what you have decided. It's a good idea to inform some close friends and relatives about your choice and how you have come through your crisis. You may have been telling people about your infertility problems all along, or you may have kept your infertility a secret. In either case, going public with your decision is a way of creating a strong sense of closure, a well-earned end to your life crisis.

Registering your decision is an act of validation. You are declaring it as valid for you. We must warn you, however, that you may not find validation from others. After we had explained our childfree decision to one of our relatives, he said to us as we were leaving, "Don't worry. You'll end up with a baby one of these days." And we have heard many stories from people who have announced their decision to live childfree to the members of their infertility support groups and have been surprised to find not validation but resistance. Some people misinterpret the childfree decision as giving up hope and have a difficult time accepting that. We have found that this is especially true among other infertile couples who may feel threatened by your getting off the infertility roller coaster. What they don't understand is that the decision to live childfree is not giving up hope but finding hope once again, the hope that you can have a good life without children.

In addition to registering your decision, another way of committing yourself to your decision is to invest yourself in it. This is a long-term activity that means, essentially, beginning to live out the decision. For us, the most powerful sign of this investment was starting to use birth control again. This had the effect of affirming that we were no longer infertile. It was a way of giving up the futile hope that somehow the period would not come. It freed us from all that. And it meant that making love became making love again, and not just trying to make babies.

The most important part of investing ourselves in our decision was acting on the positive potential it gave us. Living childfree means more than just recognizing the potential gain in your loss but making that gain a reality. We found that all the energy that had been sucked away by being infertile was released to be applied in other directions, toward work, hobbies, friends, church, families, community service, and writing this book. We invested ourselves in our decision to be childfree by acting on the opportunities that being childfree offfered. We committed ourselves to a future without children because we found that this was for us a good future, one that we wanted.

The best way to end this discussion of choice is to look at the story of how another couple made their choice to live childfree. Anne Smith tells of her infertility problems with "empty sac" syndrome which led to a series of miscarriages, the last of which was the most difficult to deal with:

This miscarriage was much harder for both of us emotionally. A decision had to be made. Our options were to try again, adopt or choose childfree with permanent birth control. The first option was ruled out. We looked to adoption, but it just didn't seem right for us because of the waiting time, cost, our age, and laws of Virginia. That seemed to only leave the childfree option.

In making this decision I had to decide what was most important to me in life. Did it have to be motherhood? Being Christian, our faith in God was most important in our decision. Through reading and prayer I believed that God has purposes for some of us other than being parents.

At this point I began to accept the childfree decision and to feel at peace with it. I knew that my husband felt the same way. This decision was made after much careful thought and many hours of talking together—not overnight. In order to be released from the bondage of infertility we needed an act of closure. Tubal ligation seemed to be the only answer. I cried for three days after signing the consent forms, but then the acceptance and contentment came to me. I began to feel good about my life and myself.

In making the childfree decision you shouldn't think of what you don't have, but what you can have. Opportunities will be available to you that you may never have dreamed of. Our decision has provided my husband and me an even greater opportunity for work in the church. I also enjoy working in my garden, watching my flowers grow and bloom. Also, my pets, a dog and rabbit, provide a lot of love, joy and happiness for me.

We offer this long quote because Anne Smith's story illustrates so well the things we have been talking about. The Smiths made the decision to be childfree by basing it on what was important in their lives. The decision was made after a lot of time and talking. They commited themselves to the decision by having a tubal ligation, which got them off the cycle of hope and despair. And most importantly, they have invested themselves in their choice by acting on the opportunities that being childfree has offered them.

6. The One Great Principle of Making Life Decisions

We've talked a lot about making life decisions in this chapter, but there is one crucial point that we haven't addressed, a point that makes life decisions easier to make. Rubin says that in the kind of decision we are talking about, there is no such thing as absolute right or wrong. What this does is free us from worrying about doing the wrong thing or the right thing.

The problem is that most people confuse life decisions with *moral* decisions. With moral decisions there *is* a right and a wrong. Moral decisions are difficult to make because they require that we choose the *right* alternative—right in the larger sense of ethical. Moral decisions, then, are ethical because they imply an absolute right or wrong.

Lewis B. Smedes, a theologian who specializes in ethics, elaborates on the difference between ethical questions and life decisions. Morality concerns "how we treat people, including ourselves. Treating people unfairly and unlovingly—this is what moral wrong is." "But," he says, "most of the time we maneuver our way through freedom zones where what matters is not whether we have done the right thing, but whether we acted wisely and well considering the options we had. There are huge areas in our lives where the question is not whether we did right or wrong, but only whether we acted like responsible people."

For us, this is a liberating concept because it frees us from the (sometimes paralyzing) fear of doing something wrong. The great thing about working in these "freedom zones" is that there is no right and wrong. There are no absolute standards to search for and thus no fears of making the wrong choice. The primary criterion for these kinds of decisions is whether it is right for you, whether it feels comfortable, whether it fits, and, as Smedes says, whether it comes of acting wisely and well. This means that we must work hard at listening and talking and respecting each other's needs. A good decision is a mutual decision.

Perhaps the most important thing that this great principle does is to underline the value of making life decisions. The value lies not in choosing the *right* alternative. No, the value is simply in *choosing*. What is important is not *what* you choose but *that* you choose. The most valuable point of this chapter is that decisions provide us a way of establishing control over our lives. It is through our decisions that we define who we are—human beings who are free to make choices about the way we live.

In matters of infertility, this idea of choice is especially helpful. Infertility robs us of the control we have over our bodies and our lives. It takes away our ability to reproduce. During the workup and the treatment, we are constantly reminded of our lack of control. Making a decision is a way of taking the wheel again. And it doesn't matter what you decide, as long as you decide.

Many people have a hard time with this concept, probably because they were raised to believe that there is a right side and a wrong side to every choice. Their greatest fear is that they will choose wrong and will regret their decision later when they find out that it was wrong. We will look at the fear of regret in Chapter Five. But for now, let us leave it that the power in making a life decision is that it commits you to something, and it is this commitment that makes it right.

7. Conclusion

One of the most painful parts of infertility is the hopelessness that people feel when they think they don't have any choices. Susanna sent us a letter that captures that hopelessness:

My husband and I are probably going to be living

child-free but not really because we choose to. We are just having to resign ourselves to having no options. We have been struggling with unexplained infertility for over 6 years, and the specialist I saw recently for a second opinion could not find anything even marginally wrong with us, so he is not even going to try any treatment. At our ages adoption of an infant would be impossible so we have not looked into that alternative. We are still trying on our own, but I have no reason to expect it to work.

What Susanna and her husband (and many other infertile couples) don't see is that there is a choice. In their resignation, they have written off adoption without even investigating it. And they conceive of childfree as having *no options.* They are stagnated and need some help to discover what their options really are.

One of the first steps to becoming childfree is to understand that living childfree is a choice. In fact, we have argued in this chapter that to be childfree you must *choose* to be childfree. It is in the act of making a decision that you gain control over your life and free yourself from your infertility.

We don't want to give the impression, though, that the three tasks of making a life decision can be done quickly. No, they take time and work. Months or even years. But it's time well spent and work that has its rewards. In the next chapter we will talk about the kind of work that is more specifically related to making the life decision to be childfree.

●

Choosing to Live Childfree

The quality of life changes dramatically once you make a definite choice. While you're still going through the frustration of trying for pregnancy or adoption, it's hard to imagine life without children as anything other than never-ending misery. But once you've decided, your energy is freed to begin making a new and enjoyable life for yourself.

—Lynne Wood

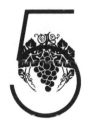

In the last chapter, we applied Dr. Rubin's ideas about decision making to the life decisions of infertility. Much of what we talked about was pretty general. In fact, a lot of it could apply to making *any* life decision. In this chapter we will focus on several issues that are more specifically related to the decision to live childfree.

It should be clear by now that for us, choice is the most important ingredient in living childfree. But just as we discovered in our research on grief, childfree is not unusual in its reliance on choice. This is an important point because it shows that childfree is not a strange state that only a few can achieve. The successful conclusion of most other life problems is also a matter of choice. The power in decision making is the peculiarly human power of taking responsibility for our lives.

We are not, then, recommending childfree as *the* resolution for infertility. We are, however, advocating the power of choice in matters of infertility. This power is especially beneficial to infertile people because we often feel like we are victims of fate with no control over our destiny. We can reassert the responsibility for ourselves through choosing, whatever the choice may be.

In this chapter, we will try to answer some questions that may have been raised by our discussion of life decisions. If having a baby has always been a life goal, is there any way you can still redefine your goals to live childfree? What does it mean to work at decision making? What is the relationship between adoption and childfree? Will making a decision take the loss away forever?

1. Redifinition: Looking at Why You Want to Have Children

In the last chapter we suggested that one approach to redefinition is to study your priorities to determine how they stack up against having children. But for some people this might not be helpful. You may find that your priorities still revolve around having a baby. This is fine unless there is some aspect of your adoption options that you can't accept. Does this mean that you are stuck in a miserable situation for the rest of your life? Not necessarily. In this section we will look at other possible ways of redefining your life.

Instead of looking for priorities outside of parenthood, this different approach asks you to look at the goals you may have for having children and then to find ways that you can reach those goals by other means. As a guide to this task we use an article by Ellen Sue Stern who explores the various needs that often lie behind the desire to get pregnant. Your reaction to this may be, "But I want to have a baby because babies are wonderful." If you are honest with yourself, though, you will probably recognize yourself in one or more of Stern's descriptions. The point of this exploration is to find a basis for redefining your life, to give you a way to change childless into childfree.

Stern says that one thing that motivates people to have children is the desire to change their lives. The changes that could result from getting pregnant are many. A woman might want to get out of the rat race and fantasizes instead about long, delicious afternoons at home with her baby. Perhaps another hoped-for change is that having a child will bring your spouse closer, spark a little more interest in your marriage. Maybe the change would be in the eyes of others. Women may dream about all the attention they will get by being pregnant or having a new baby. Men may imagine the pride that they feel announcing to the people at work that they are going to have a baby. Or maybe it is that you want your parents to think of you as an adult.

The desire to make a change in your life is probably a worthy one, and getting pregnant could certainly bring changes, though not always the ideal ones that we fantasize. But if such a desire, even in your fantasies, sparked your interest in having a child, then it's important to recognize that. It could be very helpful in deciding what course to take after infertility. Perhaps it is an indication that you could accomplish such a change by other means. Maybe what you need is to change jobs, or even to move to another city. Or maybe you should do something that you have always dreamed of doing but never seemed to find the motivation. You could take advantage of living childfree to make an important, even daring, change in your life.

According to Stern, another reason that people give for having a baby is the desire for greater stability. Some people want to put down roots, to feel like they belong somewhere, and having children can give you that feeling of the stability you remember from your own childhood in a place where you and your family belonged, or, if you don't have such memories, the stability you have found in your "Leave it to Beaver" fantasies. You may feel that your house is just not a home and that you are not a real member of a community unless you have children. If you find that this is what prompted you to want children then you may want to explore other ways of gaining that stability without children. You could join groups that benefit the community. You could get more involved in city or county activities. Become an active member of a church or synagogue. Get to know the people in your neighborhood and organize neighborhood activities. There are many ways to gain the stability of roots in a community.

Stern's third reason is a very powerful one—the longing to nurture. Most of us have enjoyed imagining what it would be like to have children to nurture, to watch them grow, to have the satisfaction of helping them mature and learn. Women may imagine helping children with their first words and finding that the first word sounds a lot like "Mommy." Men may dream of helping children with their homework or taking them to ballgames. Whatever the image is, many of us want to have children because of our craving to nurture.

What do you do with these powerful feelings if you aren't able to have children? One positive approach is to turn them outward. There are many needs in the world for the nurturing abilities that you offer. Many people volunteer for nurturing activities. And one of the advantages of this approach is that you can *choose* the age group of children and the nurturing activity that interests you most. You can become a leader in the Scouts or a youth group at your church or synagogue or join Big Brothers/ Big Sisters. You can become much more involved with children of relatives and friends. You might even find that your desire to nurture is very satisfyingly spent on plants and animals. Perhaps a strong desire to nurture might lead to a new job that offers more nurturing possibilities than your present job.

Living childfree presents many ways that you can act on your nurturing needs. For example, Lynne Wood found that being childfree left her no lack of nurturing opportunities. "As for kids," she said, "we're very involved in extended families. We're very close to the children of our closest friends and to our nieces and nephews. The interesting thing about this is that we never consciously decided to get involved to fill a void. When I started really considering childfree living, I realized that I was *already* meeting my need to nurture, and Phil was, too, by these extended family involvements."

Finally, Stern says that some people want to have a baby as a way of giving purpose and meaning to their lives. Having a child can be a way of finding a sort of immortality, a way of joining the reproductive cycle of the earth. It can be a kind of spiritual expression, an act of faith in the future of human existence. The desire for such purpose and meaning can be a very strong one. If this is one of the reasons that made you want to have children, you may despair of finding any other way to achieve your ambitions. Certainly, having children is a way to join in the cycle of creativity, but we think that there are other ways as well, ways that are perhaps even more demanding and more satisfying. You may be able to express your creativity by writing, by playing a musical instrument, by painting, by building furniture, by inventing a machine, etc. Perhaps part of the transformation from childless to childfree could be the advantage of more time and energy for your creativity.

Diane Clapp tells the story of how her miscarriage left her feeling like she couldn't create anything. "I decided then," she says, "in that dark time in my life, to do something to create something out of nothing." So she bought an old potter's wheel, took lessons, and began to make pots.

The clay felt like it would never yield to my desire

to create something from it. This stiff grey mass spinning and spinning on my wheel challenged me; I worked for hours and days. I felt the frustration and anger of infertility filtering into my experience as I struggled to create something and couldn't! On occasions I would also feel breathless with excitement as a lopsided pot emerged from the clay.

Soon I was able to pick and choose, to throw away the pots I didn't like . . . Gradually I took some power back, back from the clay and spinning wheel. My hands were in control now, they molded and formed new and beautiful shapes. I felt delight, renewed vigor and a glimmer of my "old" self . . . I was creating something that would last. The pots were never perfect and never the way I expected (or hoped) they would be. But now I can look around my kitchen and see the bowls and teapots, or feel this warm mug in my hand, and remember the pain and frustration that led me to the clay. It was a healing experience for me.

We certainly don't want to imply that living childfree is simply a matter of finding baby substitutes. As long as it's defined in terms of a substitute it cannot really be childfree. We prefer to see it more as a redefinition, an opportunity for taking the positive things a baby could bring and achieving those positive things in other ways. If you can make this leap of redefinition, childfree becomes an occasion for making good things happen in your life.

2. The Real Work of Deciding to Live Childfree: Communication

One of the features that distinguishes the acceptance of childlessness from the choice to live childfree is the amount of work that goes into achieving each. Acceptance comes quite naturally if you don't deny the loss; it's mainly a matter of time and endurance. The transformation to childfree, however, requires a conscious effort—the work that goes into making decisions.

Much of that work is communication. It's a fact: real decisions depend on real communication. To understand what this statement means, though, we need to look more closely at what communication really means.

The most popular theory of communication is what we might call the bucket theory. According to this theory, words are like buckets: we put our thoughts into them and give our thoughts to someone else. Words are simply what we use to relay what we think. The problem with the bucket theory is that it suggests that we must always know what we want to say before we say it. That puts terrible pressure on the communicator and turns talking into a process of simply stating positions. And this is not a good way to make a mutual decision.

We think of communication in a different way. Instead of using words as a way of transferring ideas, we understand communication as a way of finding out what you think, of working out your ideas *as you talk.* Communication is a way of figuring out what you mean, not just transferring ideas from one person to another. It is how you *find out* what you think, what you want, what your values are, why you fear something, etc. We prefer to see communication not simply as an act of transmission but more akin to its sister concept *communion*—a sharing of ideas, a working together to find understanding.

All this may sound too theoretical, but there are several practical advantages to viewing communication in this light. When you understand it as a way of exploring ideas, you are free to really communicate. You can say what you are thinking and feeling without fearing that you will be pinned to that position forever. You should not be like two debators who have specific positions to defend no matter what. Exploratory talking allows you simply to try out ideas, to see how they feel, to see if they fit. If they don't, then you can try out some others.

Defined this way, communication also frees the other person in the conversation. If you are talking to someone and he knows that your ideas are tentative and exploratory, more an attempt to find out what you think than to state an unequivocal position, then he is less apt to be threatened by the discussion. As a partner in the conversation, your listener's job is to help you in your search for ideas and feelings, to help you find out what you think. Using language this way means that it is a shared and sharing proposition.

A couple's decision to live childfree (and most other infertility decisions, too) must be communal. It cannot be a matter of one person imposing something on the other nor of one person putting the burden of choice on the other. It is this communal act of decision making that is the real work of the childfree choice because it is only through communication that you can come to a decision.

Our name for the communication that goes with making life decisions is *crisis communication*, to distinguish it from more casual kinds of communication. Here are five guidelines you can follow to make your crisis communication more effective.

1. It's okay to feel ambivalent. Technically, ambivalence is the feeling of being drawn in two opposite directions at once. Or more simply, it is what you feel when you don't really know what to do, when you can't make up your mind. The issue of living without children will raise ambivalent feelings. That's inevitable. After all this time *trying* to have children you are now considering *not* having children. Any major life decision—precisely because it is a major life decision—is likely to generate ambivalence.

The important thing to understand is that ambivalence is okay. And to a certain extent, it is beneficial. Unfortunately, however, a lot of people feel uncomfortable with ambivalence. Perhaps they think that not knowing what to do is a sign of weakness. Or they may assume that there is always a right way and a wrong way at every crossroads of life and if they can't find the right way they will just stay where they are.

We think that there is a more productive way to deal with ambivalence. Basically, ambivalence is nature's way of saying that it's time to talk things out. The trouble is that a lot of people run from their ambivalence. They cut off communication and with it the possibility for making a decision. Running from ambivalence simply abdicates to someone else the responsibility for making a decision. And if it's not your decision you can gain nothing from it.

2. Don't rest on assumptions. Don't assume that you know what your spouse thinks about infertility. In an article in a

RESOLVE newsletter, the Reverend Mr. John Van Regenmorter cites some interesting statistics that underline the necessity for this rule. Though most of the infertile people who were surveyed reported that they had always expected to have children, many more women than men (58% to 32%) said that they felt they were missing out on an important life goal if they didn't have children. Also, among infertile couples there was a vast difference between the way men and women felt about their infertility. Though 57% of the women said it was the hardest thing they had ever faced in their lives, only 12% of the men stated that. In addition, women reported feeling guilt and anger over their infertility much more often than men. Also, women were much more likely to report feelings of loneliness, incompleteness, helplessness, and sexual inadequacy than men.

Van Regenmorter used these statistics as a way of understanding what had happened in his own experience with infertility. His wife had assumed that he felt the same way about their infertility that she did. And he, of course, had assumed the same about her feelings. This misunderstanding of each other's feelings led to a lot of distress, particularly on his wife's part, because she then assumed that he was simply being callous and unhelpful, leaving her to suffer by herself.

It is so important not to assume what the other person is feeling. The trouble is that making such assumptions is perfectly natural: we tend to see the world through our own perspective. This is especially true when what we encounter in our spouse is a kind of grim silence, either from guilt or pain or confusion or whatever. Such silence is bound to be misinterpreted. It invites the other person to think that you are feeling the same that she is.

Communication keeps us from having to make assumptions. You should begin by accepting the fact that it's okay to feel different about your infertility. Neither party should be condemned for feeling too much nor for feeling too little. The important thing is to try to understand how you feel and why and accept the differences. You will find that understanding the differences goes a long way toward bridging those differences.

3. Be honest—and forgiving. Honesty is better than eloquence. This doesn't mean that you can't be both honest and eloquent, but sometimes when you are concentrating on making a point brilliantly and persuasively, the point becomes artificial.

It's important to remember, though, that honesty doesn't necessarily constrain you to telling only what you know is true. Usually in this kind of communication, there is no absolute truth; in fact, the point of talking is exploration, not pinning down ultimate truths. Honesty primarily means that you are honest with yourself—you say what you think you feel and not what you think you *ought* to feel.

A message about honesty particularly for men: One thing we have noticed as we have talked to people about infertility problems is the degree to which men consider it a woman's problem and tend to respond in terms of "Whatever you want, dear." This is not honest communication. This is not decision making. Instead, it is abdicating the responsibility for making a decision. Men must realize that infertility is a problem for both of you. You each must have your say in what happens. Abdicating to your wife the responsibility for making the decisions is no way to exert control over your life. Men have feelings, too, and it's dishonest to deny those feelings.

In fact, another way to interpret the radical difference between men and women in the results that Van Regenmorter cited is not that men feel any less than women but that they aren't willing to recognize those feelings. It's time for men to liberate themselves from the stereotype that society has created and to deal with their feelings. Infertility affects men, too. And if you are to gain anything in the transformation that decision making can offer, you need to be a part of that process. You need to learn how to communicate honestly, not with a goal of winning, but with a goal of exploration, not in terms of hard facts, but in terms of finding out what you feel.

Honesty also demands a willingness to forgive. In crisis communication, forgiveness means two things. First, it has the normal meaning of pardoning your spouse for things said (and done) under the trying circumstances of a crisis. This is a difficult time for both of you, and certainly no time for holding grudges or for sulking. The second meaning has to do with the exploratory nature of crisis communication. Because the purpose of this kind of communication is to try on ideas, you must make allowances. You cannot hold yourself or your spouse to an idea. Be forgiving of changes, of inconsistencies, of equivocations, of qualifiers. They are all a part of searching for an identity, of trying to define yourselves.

4. Communicate in such a way that everyone wins and no one loses. The goal of crisis communication is to build a foundation for living, and such a foundation cannot be built on the basis of winning and losing. The main threat to achieving this ideal comes from taking and defending positions. Here are some things to remember to keep from turning your communication into a massacre.

First, there is no absolute, no right and wrong. All positions are equally right and equally wrong, depending on their context. Second, the goal of your communication is to bridge gaps, to arrive at a decision that feels good to both of you. You can't do this by digging into positions. Third, if you find yourselves dug in, you should use your communication skills to understand what the other person's position is and why he or she holds that position. The key to this is listening, really listening, and putting the other position in as sympathetic terms as possible. Fourth, look for compatible feelings and ideas and use these as a basis for building something you both can agree on. And fifth, don't be afraid to change your mind. It's a sign not of a wishy-washy nature but of intelligence, the ability to see things from different perspectives.

5. Allow for lots of time. Building understanding doesn't usually happen quickly. Understanding yourself takes long enough and understanding someone else takes even longer. You don't say to your spouse, "Okay, let's sit down and hammer this thing out right now and get it over with." The pressure would be terrible. Making a major life decision takes months or even years.

One reason it takes so much time is that decision making is not an entirely rational process. Sure, you can sit down with the list of priorities and rank them from 1 to 10. You could make extensive lists of pros and cons. You can search the libraries for more information to add to your data base. But eventually a decision will just have to feel right, which seems to happen unconsciously. And that takes time.

A friend of ours, a psychologist who specializes in marital counseling, says that he uses a two-part method for helping his patients to make difficult life decisions. The first part is logical. He helps them use brainstorming techniques for generating ideas and lists of priorities and then guides them through a rational consideration of what these ideas and lists reveal. After several sessions of this careful deliberation, he then asks his patients to throw it all out and work with their intuitions, feelings and emotions. The patients then make their decision based on the way they feel, but this is inevitably colored by all the logical reasoning that they have done, too. In fact, our friend says that making a major life decision demands both sides of the person, the logical and the emotional.

The real work of the childfree life decision occurs as communication, looking at options, finding and dispensing with decision blockers, discussing priorities and values, redefining your lives according to your values, and commiting yourselves to your decision. It's a lot of work, but it's worth it. The good news is that making life decisions is a skill, and like other skills it benefits from practice and experience. Counselors say that the way you make one life decision influences the way you make later ones. You have the opportunity now to start making life decisions in a way that helps you to make them more effectively in the future. But if you find yourselves having communication problems, don't hesitate to get some help from a counselor. Communication is their specialty.

3. The Relationship Between Adoption and Childfree

Many couples we have talked to assume that the decision to stop being infertile rests simply on a choice between adoption and childfree. In fact, whenever we give our talk on choosing to live childfree, one question that invariably comes up is why we didn't adopt. We always feel uncomfortable with this question and don't quite know how to respond. On one level, we are uncomfortable because our decision not to adopt was highly personal and highly intuitive, not the sort of thing we can clearly explain to ourselves much less to anyone else. On another level, though, we feel uncomfortable with this question because it implies a confusion about the relationship between adoption and childfree.

One confusion is that childfree means finding good reasons not to adopt. We didn't see it that way at all. Adoption is a wonderful way to end your infertility crisis. We rejoice with our many friends who are happy adoptive parents. Childfree doesn't mean anti-adoption.

Another confusion inherent in the why-not-adopt question is the implication that adoption is the next natural step after infertility and that not adopting is an aberration. This confusion is certainly understandable. Infertile couples tend to develop a child fixation. Any time you want something and are not allowed to have it, you want it all the more. This is especially true when you are required to prove how much you want a child by suffering "trial by infertility treatment." So after stopping treatment the next logical step seems to be to go to the adoption agency.

A more insidious drive to adopt is the guilt of feeling selfish, that somehow not to adopt is a selfish act. Diana Burgwyn found that infertile couples often feel a subtle yet powerful pressure to adopt—a pressure that comes from within themselves as well as from others. The message they receive is that if they really wanted a child, they would adopt one. The idea is that the infertile couple who does not choose to adopt is selfish and doesn't *deserve* to have a child of their own genes.

This is, of course, irrational thinking, but sometimes it is our irrational thoughts that are the most powerful. Let's try to be rational about this for a moment. First, it's difficult to label as selfish any couple who has been through an infertility workup and treatment. Selfish people just don't make such sacrifices of health and career and social convenience.

Some couples start to feel selfish by torturing themselves with images of all those children out there who are desperately waiting for someone to adopt them. The truth is, of course, a far cry from that image. It's becoming more and more difficult to find the most frequently demanded kind of children—white infants with no mental or physical handicaps. Just ask anyone who's tried. But what about the "special" children, those who are older, retarded, racially mixed, handicapped? What if you feel guilty for not adopting one of them? Patricia Johnston says that there are about 100,000 such "special needs" children awaiting adoption. But she also says that social workers generally prefer to place them in homes with experienced parents and other children, an environment that is more conducive to their special needs.

It's okay not to adopt. You don't have to make elaborate justifications for not wanting to adopt. You are not under any obligation to explain to anyone why you don't adopt. If, after exploring the issue, it doesn't feel right to you, then don't do it.

Furthermore, adoption is not the natural next step after stopping treatment. No, adoption should be a result of choice, too; if you adopt a child it should be because you *want* to *adopt* a child. An adopted child should never be seen as a substitute for the biological child you can't have. Adoption requires that you grieve for the loss of your imagined biological child, to give up that image, and then to accept another child as your own without resentment and without always contrasting the adopted child's behavior with what your "real" child would have done. As we have been saying all along, a choice is an affirmation, not an obligation or a substitution. This affirmation is just as important with adoption as it is with being childfree.

A final confusion represented in the why-not-adopt question is that not adopting is the same thing as choosing to live childfree. As you can probably guess, we strongly disagree with that assumption. For us, living childfree is the result of an act of choice, an act of will. It is a decision to do something positive with your life. It cannot be the result of a decision *not* to do something else. The decision not to adopt may lead you to consider living childfree, but it is not itself the decision to live childfree.

In fact, we believe that neither adoption nor childfree should be a default decision. Adoption shouldn't be a substitution for a biological child. Childfree cannot be simply not adopting. Both should be the result of grieving for a loss, accepting that loss, and transforming the loss into an affirmation: either embracing someone else's biological child as your own or seizing the positive potential of living without children. We will talk more about the affirmation of adoption in Chapter Eight.

4. Reconciliation

Our experience with infertility and our research for this book has taught us a lot about loss. We've learned that grief is the natural human response to the stress that comes with loss. But we've also learned that within every loss is the potential for gain. And it strikes us as true that the greater the loss, the greater the potential gain. This is an extraordinarily hopeful view of life and of the losses that are inevitable in living. Finally, we've learned that the way to achieve the potential gain is to make a choice, to establish control over our lives again.

We don't want to leave the impression, though, that transforming loss into gain means making the loss go away forever. Another thing we have learned is that the act of choosing means embracing both the loss and the gain. Deciding to live childfree is not a magic potion that takes the painful loss of fertility and makes it disappear. We still have and probably always will have sad moments when we remember our dreams of children or have experiences we would like to have shared with a child. Choosing to accentuate the gain doesn't mean completely losing the loss.

Dr. Rubin, in another book, addresses this issue as what he calls the myth of resolution. For him and for most other people, the term resolution carries with it connotations of the eradication of conflict, the restoration of perfect internal harmony. Resolution implies an absolute state in which all division is gone.

As complex as human beings are, though, this kind of resolution is certainly an unrealistic expectation. Rubin prefers instead to use the term reconciliation, which means living in relative peace with the conflicting forces in our lives. For us, this idea of reconciliation is a good way of describing what happens in the childfree decision. Childfree doesn't mean that you are liberated forever from feelings of loss. Instead, it means recognizing that there *is* the possibility for gain and, moreover, that it is through loss that we find the gain. It means becoming big enough to embrace both the loss and the gain.

This idea of the reconciliation that comes with being childfree is illustrated by Carol Frost Vercollone's account of her visits to the card shop:

> I have gotten teary at times at card stores, and always feel at least a pang as I see the cards I'll never need. "To a precious daughter," "For our son," "To an adorable granddaughter." I have spent some painful

time in those aisles. Then I try to refocus on the sister cards and on the niece and nephew cards. And my family, equally involved in giving their earnings to Hallmark, searches out wonderful cards for Rob and me. We get beautiful cards: "For a special aunt," "For a fun uncle," but most movingly of all, cards for godparents on Mother's Day and Father's Day.

It's overly optimistic to think of childfree as a kind of antibiotic that will completely cure you of all feelings of loss. That kind of thinking is unrealistic. What childfree does is put the loss into perspective. It's okay to feel the loss because it is through the loss that we can find the gain.

5. Conclusion

For us, the key to living childfree is choice. But, as we said at the beginning of this chapter, choice is the key for resolving most life problems. There is really no mystery here: choice is a way of exerting control, and we tend to feel much more satisfied with aspects of our lives over which we have some control.

In these last two chapters we have offered some principles for guiding you toward making the choices surrounding infertility, including the choice to live childfree. These principles suggest a positive process for making those decisions. This is only a possible process, of course, because it cannot account for individual differences. But this is, very briefly, what that process looks like:

1. You begin with a need, a need for something better, and a hope that you can find joy in life again. Also important at the beginning is an awareness that choice is possible, that childfree is possible.

2. You search yourself for any decision blockers and work to reduce or eliminate them. It is necessary to grieve for and accept the loss of your fertility before you can work on living childfree. But even with acceptance of the loss, there are other blockers that could obstruct your decision making.

3. Then you do the real work of making a choice. You communicate. And through communication you search out ways to redefine your life according to the potential gains to be found in living without children. You try on the idea of living childfree and see how it fits.

4. If you find that living childfree feels right, you commit to it by registering the decision and living out the benefits that childfree offers.

●

But What About...?

For aye to be in shady cloister mew'd,
To live a barren sister all your life,
Chanting faint hymns to the cold fruitless moon.
—Shakespeare

We've given a lot of talks to various groups about living childfree. And we've noticed that after we've told our story and after we've talked about what childfree means, about grief, and about the importance of choice—in other words, when we have arrived at the 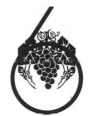 point where we are now in this book—we are always asked what we call "but what about" questions. These are very good questions that express the deep-down fears of people who face the prospect of living without children.

There must be a universal quality about these questions. We faced them ourselves as we talked about being childfree and so, clearly, have many others. It's important, then, that we deal with these questions in this discussion of living childfree; it's difficult to be truly childfree when you still have these unvoiced fears lurking in the basement or darker closets of your soul. We won't be able to completely lay them to rest here, but we hope that it may be valuable to bring them out in the open for some air. And perhaps in the light of day they may seem less fearsome.

1. But What About Regret?

"But what about regret? Won't I someday look back and regret not having children—someday when it's too late?"

Yes, regret, or rather the fear of regret, is an always menacing specter, standing out there in the future somewhere, waiting to do us in. Surely every couple who considers living without children fears that they will regret the decision. We have an image of ourselves, long past the time when any adoption agency would even talk to us, far too old for a last heroic medical effort, suddenly realizing that this was all a big mistake.

Okay, let's look at regret from another, and less threatening, angle. Everything we do brings with it the possibility of regret. Any of us might easily have come to regret whom we married, what career we pursued, which school we attended, what city we settled in, even the decision *to* have children. The fact is that every door we open closes about a dozen others, so the only way to avoid regret is never to do anything, anything at all. The fear of regret can paralyze us.

The interesting thing is that one of the antidotes for the fear of regret is the concept of choice that we have been talking about. As we said in Chapter Four, in these considerations there is no such thing as the Right Decision or the Wrong Decision, only decisions and abdications of decisions. The result is that, with unusual exceptions, we don't seriously regret our major life decisions. Sure, we have often wished, as we have agonized over a decision, that we could call up a Bureau of Right Answers. But the next best thing is for *us* to decide. We make our choices the best we can, with a human mixture of logic and emotion, and then we set about making the decision work, in effect, *turning it into* the Right Decision. It is this element of control over our lives that reduces the chances for regret.

In fact, it is those who *don't* make decisions, the drifters, who are most liable to regret. As we've said, it is our experience that most infertile couples who don't end up having children, either biologically or by adoption, tend to become drifters. They learn how to avoid the issue of their infertility. They ignore it, they don't talk about it, and they avoid situations that emphasize children. Often, however, they still have an underlying hope that this month the period won't come, hope that is regularly disappointed.

For us, this sort of drifting is the opposite of living childfree. Drifters are more likely to regret not making that last medical effort or not seeking out an adoption agency because they never made an active decision to be childfree. One reason that infertile people become drifters is that choosing takes work and demands a commitment. You've got to face your infertility and wrestle with it. You've got to communicate and see the world as open to possibility. You've also got to let go of the sometimes comfortable image of yourself as a victim of infertility. And all that's a little scary. It may seem easier just to drift.

Choice is the anchor that keeps you from drifting into regret. It is through choice that you come to embrace your life without children, to see it as something positive. But some people may find that their fear of regret is so strong that it paralyzes them. It keeps them from being able to make a choice. If you feel like this, you might consider "trying on" childfree for a period of time, paying close attention to how it feels. There are many more adoption possibilities than most people realize, possibilities that would enable you to adopt at an older age. This will give you time to test out your childfree decision without being stifled by the fear of regret.

Many people have come to terms with their fear of regret as Carol Frost Vercollone has:

> This fall and winter my brother-in-law Steve was battling lymphoma, and I identified so strongly with my sister Julia, facing losing him. Since he died, her children have been such a consolation and drawn her out of grief into the present and future. I've had so many feelings, but for myself the strongest feelings have been about being widowed without children. I've thought about being widowed without children later, but not sooner than my old age. If I am widowed at age 50, I will be even sadder not to have adopted two kids, because my priority of time with my spouse will be wiped out. I deal with that by accepting that *all* life is a risk of regret and I can only make choices with the information at hand.

2. But What About the Pressure to Have Children?

"But what about the pressure that society places on me to have children? Won't I feel like an outcast if I don't somehow have a child?"

Susan wrote to us about the premium placed on having children and how she and her husband feel about it. "We have enjoyed our close-knit community church for many years. This spring three of the women our age were pregnant. The entire focus of the church seemed to turn to these babies. I just could not deal with three baby showers, three rose presentations to new babies, three dedication ceremonies. We have been trying to find another church, but so far have not found one that is home to us."

Most of us know what it feels like—the subtle and not-so-subtle pressures to have babies. Distant in-laws asking, "So what's taking you so long? When are you going to start popping them out?" The barrage of Mother's and Father's Day ads. The baby showers with their focus on how wonderful it is to be pregnant. The seemingly incessant talk about children at parties. We visited some married friends once and ended up standing around a sand box—the couple, all of their parents, and us, eight adults—staring at a six month old. It almost seems sometimes that we live in a culture of child (and parent) worshippers. How can we talk of affirming a life without children in such a society?

This force that we feel has a name, pronatalism, which Diana Burgwyn defines as "an attitude or policy that exalts motherhood and encourages parenthood for all." We found it very helpful to understand more about pronatalism, particularly since our choice to live childfree seems to fly in the face of it. Two books that provide useful information on pronatalism are Burgwyn's *Childless by Choice* and Elizabeth M. Whelan's *A Baby . . . Maybe.*

It's easy to see why society should encourage parenthood and hold it up as an ideal. Throughout nature, the strongest force is the continuation of the species—stronger, often, than survival of the individual. Each human sub-group—family, nation, culture, race—does the same thing by encouraging its members to reproduce, by rewarding those who do and by guarding the next generation.

Pronatalism has been a part of human custom and law for thousands of years. Whelan reminds us that the Code of Hammurabi in Babylon, 40 centuries ago, contained laws to increase the birth rate. In Rome in the 1st century A.D., fathers with greater numbers of children got preference in public office; mothers were allowed to wear special clothes and ornaments. In other lands special tax breaks or pensions were given to parents.

In many African villages, an entire day of feasting and praise is set aside for honoring a women who has recently given birth. Religions have always encouraged procreation. The most obvious example is the Catholic Church, which forbids contraceptive technology in any form and flatly states that reproduction is the purpose of married love.

How does society communicate this mandate to us? Somehow we are all reared in the knowledge that this is what is expected of us. References to our future children start very early. A friend still laughs at her mother's angry curse: "I hope your children act just like you!" Connie told us that when she was about ten years old she asked her mother how she would ever be able to repay her for all she had done for her. Her mother's reply: "Only by doing the same for your own children some day."

The pressures and reminders are particularly strong immediately after, or even during, the wedding ceremony. The Greek Orthodox service especially is full of explicit prayers and admonitions for fertility, but the wish is at least implicit in every standard ceremony. The push from parents is particularly strong at this time. This is their payoff, the reward for their efforts, the hedge against a lonely old age. They have been led by a pronatalist society to expect this. Our favorite illustration of this is the experience of a friend of ours who borrowed his father-in-law's new car and accidently ran it into the corner of the older man's garage. Instead of the expected lecture, he was told, "It's all right, as long as you keep giving me grandchildren."

The reminders of our "duty" to reproduce come from television, newspapers, the pulpit. Mother's Day and Father's Day are yearly reminders that our nation holds parents in special esteem. Any mother can tell you of the (often too brief) moment in the sun she enjoyed around the time of the birth of each child, especially the first, as she was temporarily the center of attention. It alters her status in the family, especially her husband's family, with "the mother of my grandchildren" being considerably higher on the ladder than "my son's wife."

The force of pronatalism does not even let up after the birth of the first child. We were discussing societal pressure with a group of parents and complaining about the fact that so many people felt they had a right to comment critically on our childlessness. One by one other couples spoke up and pointed out that they too had earned unsolicited criticism for only having one child; for having six children; for waiting five years before the second child; for having two within one year. As Elizabeth Whelan says: "One peculiarity of the parenthood issue is that everyone has an opinion on a subject that is really none of his business!" And we have discovered that almost everyone feels perfectly free to express that opinion.

Of course it's difficult to be infertile in the midst of all this pronatalism. But if you can get out of your infertility for a moment, you may be able to see that pronatalism is, at its root, a good thing. In a sense, the issue of procreation *is* society's business. It is understandable that a culture would encourage its own continuation and find ways to reward and/or bribe those who are doing an important and underpaid job.

This perspective of pronatalism is extremely helpful for us. The rude comments of co-workers and acquaintances and even strangers, the hearts and flowers of Mother's Day, the baby fixations of our friends—these things aren't really, as they often seem, directed at our own incapacity to have children. They are the manifestations of pronatalism, the influence of our culture, our history, our religion, and even our government.

Knowing about pronatalism doesn't make it go away. And, indeed, we wouldn't want it to go away. It serves an important function for us all. However, knowing about it, putting a name on it, does help us to be stronger in the face of it. The decision to have children, whether biologically or by adoption, should be your own. And if you choose not to? Well, fortunately, there are other ways to make your place in your culture besides having children.

3. But What About the Maternal Instinct?

"But what about the maternal instinct? Won't I feel unfulfilled all my life if I don't have children?" (We think it's interesting that few people ever ask about the *paternal* instinct.)

In the process of trying to sort out how much of your desire for children is due to societal expectations and how much is coming from within you, you have to wrestle with the concept of maternal instinct. Is there such a thing? Is there, somewhere in your DNA, a program for parenthood that you must follow or be forever frustrated?

Some of the women who wrote to us were grappling with these questions. Frankie faced her fears that she would never be "fulfilled" or "complete as a woman" unless she experienced motherhood. Sally was surprised when she realized that her marriage was more important to her than being a mother. "Maybe this means I don't *need* to be a mother as much as I thought."

Clearly, animals have instincts that allow them to know what behaviors are appropriate for producing and nurturing their young. But these seem to be built-in instructional programs, and we don't know if they also make the animal "want" offspring, nor do we know anything about the quality of its life if it does not happen to reproduce.

Human beings are the only self-aware animal and therefore these issues are infinitely more complex. For us, continuation of the species is not the only goal that drives our lives; we also strive for other things, such as quality of life, satisfaction, and productivity and creativity of a non-biological nature. Ultimately, our survival as a race depends less on our success in replicating our genetic material than it depends on our ability to solve the military and environmental problems that we have created.

Psychologists are divided on whether human beings must bear and rear children in order to be psychologically healthy. Whelan reviews both sides of the question very well. Freud believes that we must do so, that this is how a woman deals with her penis envy. Erikson includes the rearing of children as a necessary stage in achieving maturity.

On the other extreme are more modern psychologists who repudiate any idea of innate need or desire to reproduce. Whelan quotes Dr. William Goode: "There are no instincts. There are reflexes, like eye blinking, and drives like sex. There is no innate drive for children. Otherwise, the enormous cultural pressures that there are to reproduce would not exist. There are no cultural pressures to sell you on getting your hand out of the fire."

The truth probably lies somewhere in the middle: we are

neither driven by an undeniable biological destiny nor are we brainwashed into parenthood by society. Our wish for children goes deeper than the level of rational logic, but that does not mean that we create unsolvable psychological problems if we choose a different course. Indeed, the growing number of couples who are voluntarily childfree suggests that there are many people who are now choosing a different course.

As we said earlier, most people do have strong needs to nurture, to create, to leave something behind when they are gone. Perhaps the desire to be mothers and fathers is bound up in these needs and thus not really an instinct at all. Either way, children provide a fine outlet for such needs, but they are not, we think, the only outlet. Parents and non-parents alike should look elsewhere to find ways to be nurturing, creative, and "immortal."

4. But What About Old Age?

"But what about old age? Who's going to take care of me if I don't have children?"

These questions express what seems to be the greatest fear of all. Many of us dread getting old and helpless even more than dying, imagining ourselves as lonely old people with no one to visit us or to take care of us when we are unable to take care of ourselves. This seems to be a universal fear, with people who have children not wanting to be a burden to them and people who don't have children worried that no one will care for them. There are no easy responses to these fears. But interviews with childless people give valuable insights into aging without children. Some of the information confirms that there is indeed a potential problem and some of it points to ways we can improve our prospects.

Burgwyn points to sociological studies confirming that the major social resource of the elderly in our society is their adult children. Contact with anyone who is not kin declines as health declines. When polled about their general satisfaction with life, childless people without spouses scored a little lower than parents without spouses. Another interesting difference between these two groups is that more than 83% of the former live alone, whereas only 65% of the latter do. The difference is primarily in the number living with grown children.

But these statistics only show the surface and don't indicate what individual lives are like.

Is living alone always a bad thing and always not by choice? Burgwyn cites Robert S. Brown in *The Elderly in America* who reported that 68% of elderly parents saw one of their children at least once a week but only 17% reported "close affectional ties" with them. "It is undeniable," Burgwyn says, "that children might brighten and lighten old age. But the fact that one is old and childless does not automatically guarantee a miserable old age any more than children guarantee a happy life."

The childfree people who wrote to us were unanimous in the opinion as expressed by Dwayne that "the poorest reason for having children is to have someone to take care of you in your old age." They often pointed to elderly people they knew whose children gave them no emotional or financial support. Several expressed a desire to get involved now in the lives of older people.

What, then, does enable one to be satisfied in the later years? A consistent picture emerged from our reading.

Burgwyn points out that the voluntarily childless were more content than the *in*voluntarily childless. Perhaps they engaged their lives more creatively and positively and spent less time on regrets. She also found that in studies on this subject there was wide agreement that "the childless aged who are profoundly affected by the absence of children are those whose social resources were never very ample." The childless elderly who do well seem to have built a network of support around themselves through the years. There are brothers and sisters and younger relatives or friends of all ages, or close ties with community groups, churches and service organizations. They actively pursue hobbies, work, or other interests and continue to find opportunities for learning and growing.

In addition, Merle Bombardieri, in her RESOLVE fact sheet on childfree living, points to some other factors that influence the quality of old age. Health is a major factor that we have only limited control over, but financial stability is also very important and is something we can actively work on now with early and aggressive retirement planning. She also points to assertiveness as a valuable quality. We can begin now to learn to ask for and get the help we need.

A life turned outward, concerned and involved with other people, will not suddenly collapse and become narrow in old age just because there are no children.

Burgwyn sums it up: "As a parent one tends to live with the hope that in old age the children will provide emotional and perhaps concrete support and add meaning to one's life. This may or may not become reality. But the childless have no such expectations: they know they will have to look elsewhere—to other relatives, friends, neighbors, community groups, and above all their own inner resources. How they deal in midlife with approaching old age will determine in large measure how rich, or, conversely, how impoverished those final years will be."

5. Conclusion

Living childfree means embracing your childlessness and making the most of your life without children. It is one positive response you can make to your infertility. However, it's difficult to be childfree if you feel weighed down by the fears we have been talking about in this chapter.

For us, childfree does *not* mean that these fears have been forever vanquished and we can walk blithely through life never feeling a twinge from them again. That's a foolish expectation. Instead, childfree means that we face these fears, understand where they come from, and *do* something about them. It means preparing for old age emotionally and financially. It means finding other outlets for maternal/paternal "instincts." It means understanding what pronatalism is and separating what society wants from what we want. And it means circumventing the possibility of regret by *choosing* how we will live.

In short, childfree doesn't mean that the fears vanish; it means that they become manageable.

●

The Future

When you are chasing the dream of a baby, it is easy to forget that life has the potential for many other dreams and fulfillments.

—Linda Salzer

In the preface of this book we noted that we hope to reach readers who are at different stages of their infertility journeys. One group is readers who are still early in infertility treatment, perhaps only just diagnosed. Though the odds are good that you will be able to  have children, right now you don't know. This book on living childfree offers you the hope that if you *can't* have children there is still an opportunity for a happy ending to your infertility crisis. It's not a matter of adoption or nothing. You are not condemned to an incomplete life if you don't have children. There is hope for your future.

Another group is readers who are in the middle of the infertility experience. You have exhausted most reasonable medical efforts and are trying to decide what comes next, one last medical try, adoption, or living childfree. We hope that we have been able to answer your questions about what it means to live childfree. We've tried to show that living childfree really is one way to stop being infertile. But no matter what you choose, there is hope in your future.

Or maybe you are among the group we have called drifters. You have put off doing anything about your infertility so long that it's no longer an open issue. Because you still haven't resolved your infertility, you remain childless, the emphasis in your life on what you don't have. We invite you to try to start talking again. Of course, it will hurt to reopen those old wounds, but if those wounds still haven't healed and are getting infected, it's better to open them now before the infection spreads. If you can do this, there is hope in your future, too.

As we've said before, we don't see ourselves as recommending childfree over adoption or any other way of putting your infertility behind you. However, we do recommend choice and communication, the keys to making any life decision. Childfree is only one way to resolve your infertility crisis.

Childfree, like having a child, is future oriented. It is a way of being no longer infertile, an invitation to look toward a future without children of your own. In this chapter we will take a look at the future for people who are childfree—what to expect and how to prepare for it.

1. Is Childfree Right for Your Future?

Is a childfree life right for you? We, of course, can't answer that, but we can offer one way of judging whether it is for you. First, let's look at a discussion by Jean E. Veevers about the voluntarily childless (people who are not infertile but choose not to have children), from which we will get some concepts we can apply to choosing to live childfree.

Veevers describes two groups of people who make up the voluntarily childless, the Early Articulators and the Postponers. The Early Articulators make it clear from the beginning that they don't want to have children. Their choice is mainly a negative one. But most of the voluntarily childless are Postponers, people who simply put off deciding to have children until they simply don't. They are not so much against children as in favor of other things.

Let's use these same terms and apply them to people who *want* to have children. In this case, the Early Articulators are those who have no doubts about whether they want to have children and have made their preference known before they get married. They usually try to get pregnant as soon as they are married. Postponers generally put off having children until "the time is right." Education and career, at least for a while, take precedence over having a baby. Postponers may even be ambivalent about whether they want children at all and have to make a conscious decision about it.

Our experience suggests to us that, *generally speaking,* infertile people who are Early Articulators will be less likely to choose childfree than Postponers. We have no evidence from research to prove this theory, but it does seem to make sense.

Sharon Covington, a counselor who works with infertile couples, says that there are some who are absolutely set on having children. "For many infertile couples I counsel, the idea of there being a choice involved in a life without children is incomprehensible. How can it be that after all the years of tests, treatments, and tears, a couple could choose *not* to have children? For many couples, the very thought brings up intensely negative feelings and that in itself may be a clue that it is not an option for them."

Such couples are typically not candidates for becoming childfree. They have defined their lives as parents and know exactly what they want. Because they are so focused on having children, they cannot even consider childfree as an alternative for them. That's a pretty clear indication that they should try other channels for achieving their dream.

Postponers, though, tend to be those who *can* consider childfree as an alternative to infertility. They are typically people who have, at some point in their married lives, found that there were other values that took priority over having children. We believe that Postponers are more likely to be able to rediscover those values again and perhaps even find other values that will lead them to see living without children as an opportunity instead of a curse.

Sometimes, however, it is possible to lose touch with the way we felt about having children before we were diagnosed as infertile. Linda Salzer, author of *Infertility: How Couples Can Cope*, says that "It is possible that some people are at first uncertain about becoming parents but make the effort anyway, only to be confronted with their infertility. In the process of fighting the problem, they may forget their early doubts and be drawn into a battle to regain control of their fertility—only now not so much because they desire children but because they want it to be a choice." It may take some work to figure out what your motivation really is, but what you discover will help you decide whether living childfree is for you. It is largely a matter of values and priorities, and we talked about getting reacquainted with your priorities in Chapter Four.

We don't want to imply, however, that Early Articulators

can't live childfree. Some of you may not be able to have children by any means at all, but that doesn't mean that you are destined to live child*less* all your life. It will take a lot of work to redefine your life so that you are childfree, but it can be done. "Redefinition: Looking at Why You Want to Have Children" in Chapter Five offers some guidance for doing that work. Also, a counselor can help.

But what if yours is a "mixed marriage," an Early Articulator married to a Postponer? It will probably take a lot of work to find a resolution that both of you can be happy with. And you also may need the direction a counselor can provide. Lynne Wood tells how counseling helped her and her husband.

> I wanted to adopt, but [my husband] Phil didn't. I remember our driving home from an adoption meeting and comparing reactions. While I was happily fantasizing about our adopted family, Phil was concluding that adoption was not for him. He just wasn't sure he could finally commit himself to accept and raise a child who was not his own flesh-and-blood. I was in a dilemma—how could I adopt if my husband was against it? Suddenly I was very lonely. Infertility treatment had brought us together, but the adoption issue set us at odds with each other. It was very isolating.

> We went together to a counselor who was very helpful. It turned out that I had never really let go of the hope that I would get pregnant. I had some grief work to do before I could give the childfree choice any consideration. Counseling enabled us to renew our commitment to each other and to our marriage. Only after grieving and renewing my commitment to Phil, was I ready to consider and to accept remaining childfree.

2. What to Expect from Others

We get it all the time. We meet another couple at a party and get the inevitable question, "Do you have children?" One of us will say, simply, "No, we don't." And then there is that awkward moment before we can deflect the question by asking about their children. In that moment, we can almost see it in their eyes: classification: DINKS: double income no kids. Selfish people who don't want to share their lives with children.

Unless we are pressed, we prefer not going into the details of our infertility with casual acquaintances, so their initial impression of us is often the one they keep. This jet-set perception of childless people was fueled by the September 1986 *Newsweek* cover story on the rising rate of voluntary childlessness, which pictured fast-living couples driving two-seater sports cars, eating gourmet take-out, and living in rooms with pristine white carpets. No wonder some people assume that we are selfish—guilt by association!

Of course, accusations of selfishness are particularly wrong-headed when they are leveled at people who have wanted children badly enough to go through what we have gone through. "Contrary to the stereotype of selfishness," Merle Bombardieri points out, "a high percentage of childfree people are teachers, social workers, or people who spend their weekends doing volunteer work with children or for a social cause. It's far more common for selfish, immature people to have children for selfish, immature reasons."

One way to explain the assumption of selfishness that living childfree sparks in some people is to say that they are envious of the way we live. But that is probably too simplistic an explanation. It is more likely the case that they see our choice to live happily without children as threatening. Rearing children is a tough, stressful job that requires a lot of support. This is the kind of support that pronatalism provides, and that's why it's so important to society. But the rejection of that pronatalism implied in our *not* having children may appear to undercut that support. It is surprising that in a country where the divorce rate makes you feel doomed as you leave the altar and where more than half of our school children are living in single-parent homes, the decision to make a good life without children still has the power to shock and offend. Even people who are cynical about love and marriage *still* act as if parenting were somehow sacred.

Even with sympathetic friends and relatives, it is very

difficult to get the childfree decision validated. We don't yet live in a world where differences are easily tolerated. The family myth of "Leave It to Beaver" and "Father Knows Best" still has great power for our society—breadwinning father, nurturing mother, and two or three happy children.

It can be very frustrating for a couple who has struggled, grown, and felt their way out of the pain of infertility by becoming childfree, only to be met with misunderstanding, even when it is well-meant. If a couple announces, "We are going to have a baby!" they are received with smiles and hugs and warm congratulations. When they say "We're going to have a good life without children," though, there are no feelings of triumph from friends and family. The usual response is, "I'm so sorry," or "Have you considered X adoption agency?" In the early days of the childfree life, this can be a very wounding experience, with each out-of-sync response causing you to doubt your own choice. "How can we be right when we're so different from all these couples?"

It's helpful for us to know that even when the responses of friends and relatives may hurt, they are usually prompted by only the best of motivations. They are often very happy with their own children and want us to have the same happiness. Also, to people who aren't acquainted with the long, painful, emotion-laden journey you have made, the decision to stop trying to get pregnant looks like giving up hope, something we've been taught never to accept. They are not aware that after a certain point in the infertility process hope becomes the enemy, an obstacle to forward progress.

There will be a rare few who say, "I understand what you're doing and I'll support you all I can," even if it is not what they would have decided. In dealing with the others, even friends and relatives, it is very helpful to remember that their responses have more to do with them and their problems and dreams than with you and yours. Remember, also, the long months (maybe even years) it took you to arrive together where you are now. It's not fair to expect even those who love you to understand and accept it quickly.

It is surprising, though, that sometimes even people who *are* familiar with your journey will react negatively to your decision to live childfree. We are referring specifically to fellow members of infertility support groups or counseling groups. RESOLVE, the best known national infertility support group and the one that we are most familiar with, is firm in its position that childfree is one way to resolve infertility and is very supportive of infertile couples who have made that choice.

But even within RESOLVE, this position may sometimes not be reflected in a particular support group. Sally, for instance, said, "I feel a lack of support in my decision to be childfree . . . When I was infertile I was very active in RESOLVE and that was so soothing. But one by one, people had babies or adopted. So I feel very alone." And after Margery told us that she had chosen to live childfree, she added, "Frankly, I have gotten very little support from RESOLVE members in this choice."

This is not an unreasonable response from other members of an infertility support group. People who are in the midst of an infertility treatment or a prolonged adoption process could very easily misinterpret their fellow members' decision to live childfree as giving up. For them, the purpose of the group is to help each other through the trials of infertility toward having children.

This view is certainly excusable in people who are so wrapped up in trying to get pregnant. For us, though, the purpose of infertility support groups is for members to help each other through the infertility crisis—however that crisis is resolved. It is important that members of infertility support groups understand that the childfree decision is a viable way not to be infertile anymore. It is just as good as having a child biologically or by adoption and a lot better than drifting for the rest of your life as childless. Our hope is that when former support group members gather for an alumni picnic, childfree couples will be received with the same joy as those who can show off their babies.

Here are two solutions to this problem, the first from Dan, a correspondant, and the second from Sharon Covington in her article, "Childfree: The 'Closet' Choice":

> Groups like RESOLVE are very important support groups to help infertile couples cope. They offer counseling, information on adoption, and doctors who specialize in infertility. But what about the persons who've been through all that and opt for a

childfree relationship? It seems there should be a tributary of RESOLVE emerging called "Evolved," an organization specifically for childfree couples.

What can we, as RESOLVE members, do to help the childfree couple come out of the closet? First, we have to come to terms with our own prejudices and fears about childfree living. The more open, honest, and supportive we can be to someone who has made a different choice, the more "acceptable" they will feel. Second, we can help give couples who make this choice some positive recognition for having reached a resolution. Since births and adoptions are announced in the newsletter, we could encourage a similar proclamation for the couple who has made the decision to remain childfree. Last, we need to continue to facilitate a support network within RESOLVE for couples who have chosen or are considering a childfree life like we do for adoption, A.I.D. [DI], etc.

We've talked about dealing with casual acquaintances, friends and relatives, and fellow support group members, but the most difficult encounters for most childfree couples are with their parents, whose own life plans and dreams for the future are affected by our decision. Mack and Diana didn't even tell their parents about their radical, and ultimately unsuccessful, treatments for infertility: "Our parents did not know, at least we didn't tell them, that we made an effort to give them grandchildren. We did not want to cause more pain than was necessary if it did not work out . . . We realize that there may come a day when we will share this part of our lives with them, but the time has not come yet."

After struggling to come to terms with our own disappointment, we must now face up to our parents'. This is especially hard if one of us is an only child. Many parents see grandchildren as the "pay-off" for the hard work of parenting. We need to acknowledge their disappointment and allow them to come to terms with it by making choices of their own. They may find alternative ways of grandparenting!

Beyond their disappointment, they may also genuinely feel that we are making the wrong decision. However, by this time of life, most parents have disagreed with their children before. They have had to let us be adults and solve our own problems as best we can, whether or not our solutions are the ones they would have chosen. They have learned how to support us even when they disagree with us—and if they haven't, we have learned to live without their support.

One thing we have to understand is that our parents want us to be happy, and they probably want that even more than grandchildren. This is especially true when they realize that we *can* be happy without children, that children are not the only thing that makes a marriage—or a family. If we have conscientiously decided that this is the choice for us, then all we can do is live affirmatively with it. As life becomes better for us, and as the pain of infertility recedes, it will be easier for those who love us to understand and accept.

We wish that we had done a better job of helping our parents understand our decision to live childfree. After a long and private battle with our infertility, we made a special trip to each of our homes to tell our parents that we were infertile and would not be able to bear them grandchildren. We and our parents shared tears of disappointment around the kitchen table. But it wasn't until well after that sad trip that we had worked through to our decision to live childfree. Our lives were good again, our disappointment gone, but what about our parents?

We didn't really know how to explain childfree to ourselves, much less to them. We didn't know of any information on living childfree to send them. They could tell that we were happy with our lives, but that wasn't quite enough. We wish that we had included them in our decision to live childfree by helping them to understand what it means to be childfree, by telling them the story of how we had come to that decision, by showing them that this is the way we will put our infertility behind us and get on with our lives as positively as we can. They are by necessity affected by our infertility; they should also be included in the renewed life that we have when we are no longer infertile.

We would like to be able to offer solutions for all the problems we have raised in this section: the perfect riposte to the rude inquisition of a stranger, the ideal response to overly solicitous friends, or just the way to help your family understand what you are going through. We can't do that. But we can offer you this brief discussion of *why* people respond the way they do. You can be more sympathetic—and more appropriate in *your* reactions—when you understand what motivates other people.

Though we don't have all the answers, we *can* offer the hope from our own experience that this issue will become less painful with time, as you and your circle of family, friends and acquaintances get used to the idea of your being childfree. After a little experience, questions like "Do you have children?" won't be so difficult to handle. And as you get older, the social focus on babies will begin to recede and friends may admit envy that you have no teenagers or college tuitions to worry you. When you can see your own life as an affirmation, it's difficult for others not to see it that way too, and soon the painful associations of "infertile" and "childless" will fade.

The main problem in dealing with others is, as usual, misunderstanding. We need to help other people be more aware of infertility issues in general and of the childfree resolution in particular. We hope that this book might make a contribution to the latter. In fact, one of the reasons we have written it is because we wish we had had something like it to send to people we care about so that they would understand our decision. We hope that it may be used that way by others.

3. What to Expect in Living Childfree

We've presented a very positive portrayal of the possibilities for living childfree. We thought that at this point it might be beneficial to take a look at some of the sociological studies of people who live without children. It might be good to know what we can expect.

In 1983, Jean E. Veevers, in *Contemporary Families and Alternative Lifestyles,* reviewed the sociological research on childless couples (not limited to the voluntarily childless). She discovered that there was in the general population a widespread acceptance of pronatalism and a negative perception of childless men and women. However, psychological studies on the childless found no evidence of poor mental health or lack of social or sexual adjustment. The divorce rate among the childless was not higher, contrary to the widespread notion that having children will cement a marriage. In fact, several studies found that childless persons were more likely to report their marriages as "very happy" than parents. In old-age studies, widows with children tended to be happier than those without, but if the spouse was still alive there was no difference. There was also no difference between parents and non-parents in responses to questions about loneliness, health, or general quality of life.

Research generally shows that life for the childless is not any less satisfying than for parents and can, in some ways, be better. Referring to non-parents, Marian Faux says, "Their marriages retained a special vitality and closeness that sociologists have come to associate with childless couples." Diana Burgwyn found that the marriages of childless couples tended to be characterized by high degrees of intimacy and interdependence and even preoccupation with each other. Indeed, there was a certain danger of closing out the outside world and being too vulnerable to the loss of the spouse.

Burgwyn also found that childless people often retain childlike qualities themselves, sometimes amounting to abdication of adulthood. She would often hear them say, "I don't know what I want to be when I grow up." This might require that they work harder at accomplishing adult tasks—like establishing mature relationships with their parents. But it can make them delightfully fun to be around—especially for children. The authors of *Mary Poppins, Peter Pan*, the Dr. Suess books, and *Alice in Wonderland* were all childless. As psychiatrist R.E. Gould said, "Childless people make wonderful aunts and uncles."

Childless couples don't own pets more often than parents but seem to focus their mutual attention more intensely on them. Or sometimes these couples have other things which they both personify and take care of, such as a career, a project, or a book. The idea of a child substitute is not a myth.

Carol and Robert Vercollone bear out these findings about childfree couples. Carol writes:

We joke that Rob helps us with our childlessness because he can be as playful as any kid. I guess I have no problem "getting in touch with my inner child" either. And though I hesitate to reinforce a stereotype that sometimes makes us look foolish, pets are important in our life too. I've had Leona since I was 21, longer than many other friendships, and Corky adopted us three years ago and has given up his life on the streets. Yes, we know it can be insulting or pathetic to equate them with children, but . . . they sure are a focus for nurturing and play each day.

So the picture that we secretly feared did not emerge: maladjusted people with tottering marriages living their lives with "something missing." Instead we found a pattern of rich diversity with as much potential for stability and satisfaction as any other life choice could offer.

As you get older, there are other considerations that have special significance for the childfree. People without children sometimes find that certain holidays which focus so much on children begin to lose their appeal. In our society, many religious observances, even those which in their origin had little to do with children, have become heavily associated with children: Christmas, Hannakah, Easter with its bunnies and candies, and the Seder with its role of teaching the Passover tradition to the children. You don't have to be locked into celebrating these holidays in the traditional ways. Merle Bombardieri suggests that childfree couples start some "new traditions." Some years you could take a vacation for two at Christmas or invite Jewish friends to Christmas Eve dinner. You could invite Christian friends to the Seder and let it be an education for them. You could have an Easter egg hunt in your backyard for the neighborhood children. Yours could be the place for the yearly Halloween costume party for adults after their kids have trick or treated. Put your imagination to work. It could be fun!

For a woman, menopause (or a hysterectomy) can be a particularly difficult time, as she finds it necessary to mourn her unborn children one last time. But the other side of this coin is that the end of the menses can bring with it a great sense of relief and renewal. The agony of the testing, hoping, and decision-making are finally over, and the pressures of pronatalism have been turned onto younger targets. In almost all cultures, Margaret Mead reports, there is an increase in women's creativity at this time. The middle-aged childless often find themselves better off financially than parents and can enjoy renewing friendships with parents whose children have now left home.

Another major crisis of growing into middle age is the death of one's own parents. This brings into focus one last time our failure to produce the next genetic generation, to pass on what was left to us. It also makes us face up to our own death as never before, as though a buffer between us and death had been removed.

For most people, middle age is a time to worry about our "immortality." Are we leaving a mark on the world? Has our career worked out the way we had hoped? Will we be remembered for something? Have we made a contribution that will justify our existence?

It will help to do a lot of thinking about this while we are still young. What *does* give meaning to our lives? Is it necessary for everyone to leave a major social, scientific, or artistic legacy? For most people, the longing for "immortality" is satisfied by producing children. But what about us? Do we have to be superhuman to attain this satisfaction without children? Not necessarily. Psychiatrist Robert Gould (quoted in Burgwyn) says, "A constructive, useful life, good works and good relationships are as valid as writing poetry or inventing a machine. Anything that one does well and obtains satisfaction from is a good enough reason for living. To be a decent human being that people like and feel better for knowing is enough."

Another great hurdle of middle or later life is the loss of one's spouse. This is especially traumatic for couples without children because they have a tendency to become absorbed in each other, often to the exclusion of other affections and supports. When a spouse dies, there is quite often a wish for a child as a reminder, a piece of him or her to continue in the world.

But Diana Burgwyn points out that the loneliness that occurs after the death (or even loss through divorce) of a spouse is a *specific* loneliness for *that* relationship and that even if children were present they could not fill that void. Elizabeth

Whelan quotes Lynne Caine, the author of *Widow:* "People shouldn't look to children to alleviate loneliness. I'm really fierce on this subject. It's not fair to attempt to drain them in this fashion. It can only make them feel guilty for not being able to do enough."

Whatever our future holds, we know that we go into it united on at least one thing: the decision to live childfree. We find the significance of that decision in a statement that we found in Veever's book: "The distinction between voluntary and involuntary childlessness is of paramount importance . . . Theoretically and pragmatically, the consequences of a phenomenon must be assumed to be quite different if it involves the achievement of a major life goal, or the frustration of one. 'Choice may well be one of the most significant determinants of satisfaction with a particular lifestyle.'"

This last sentence reveals a truth that is very important to us. It is choice that makes the difference between voluntary and involuntary childlessness. Childfree means turning involuntary childlessness into voluntary childlessness. And we would rather live our lives in the achievement of a major life goal than in the constant reminder of the frustration of one.

4. Making Plans for your Future

We are still relatively young and have few role models in the older generation to guide us as we look toward the years ahead without children. However, we have learned enough from our research to formulate a few guidelines to keep in mind as the time goes by.

1. Plan for your financial future. Some careful homework now and the discipline to put aside some of the money that would have been spent on children can help alleviate some of the fear of financial hardship in old age. Of course money won't buy love and companionship, but it can buy food, shelter, and health care and can keep us independent a little longer.

2. Plan early where you will retire. Go to work well ahead of time to establish contacts and involvement there. It doesn't make sense for a childless couple to spend a lifetime establishing a network of friends, interests, and activities in one

town and then move to a condo in Florida at age seventy.

3. Plan now for immortality. Decide early whether it is important to you to leave a lasting mark on something. Figure out, if you can, what constitutes a good enough justification for your life. Don't wait until you're sixty-eight to realize you really wanted to be an African missionary. Be one now.

4. Turn yourself outward. Resist the temptation to become wrapped up in yourselves as a couple. Seek out contacts of all kinds that might widen your circle of human interaction. The gifts you have to offer won't travel out of your home on the feet of your children; you'll have to carry them out yourself.

5. Sweet Grapes; Or, Here's to the Future!

We began this book by telling the story of our infertility. Everybody who has faced infertility has a story to tell. The stories have a common theme in the pain, fear, loneliness, bitter disappointment, and confusion that accompanies infertility. But most of these stories have happy endings. Most couples eventually get the biological child they wanted. Some can tell of the success of medical miracles such as in vitro fertilization. Others adopt a child who becomes their own.

Another happy ending to an infertility story comes when a couple makes the decision to live childfree. In fact, we believe that deciding to live childfree is just as successful a conclusion to an infertility crisis as getting a baby. It's not giving up or taking what's left—the booby prize. It is the hard-won decision to transform the loss of fertility into gain for our lives, to change sour grapes into sweet grapes.

The title of this book, of course, is a reversal of the Aesop's fable in which the fox, after trying in vain to snatch some grapes just out of reach on a vine overhead, slinks away muttering, "I bet they were sour anyway." For us, that fox represents people who are embittered by what they can't have. Some, like the fox, turn their bitterness on the grapes and declare them not worth having in the first place. They refuse even to talk about it, and their bitterness seeps out into their homes. For others, those grapes only become sweeter and sweeter as they pace in circles under them, hoping that one might drop. They begin to define their whole lives as sour in contrast to the wonderful sweetness of those grapes, which they can never reach.

We want to offer another alternative. We know that those grapes are sweet and will be a tasty treat for whoever can reach them. But we also know that on other vines there is other fruit that is just as sweet and within our reach.

That is the fruit that will sustain us.

●

Open to Adoption: Considerations of Traditional Adoption, DI, Surrogacy, and Embryo Transplant

No child should grow up being considered second best. Every child deserves a family that loves her for herself because of the special person she is.

—Joan McNamara

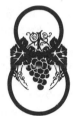

Here's an optimistic perspective on infertility: being infertile gives us the opportunity to really explore our reproductive lives and to choose options that others typically don't even consider. In a way, the loss of control over our fertility gives us *more* control over our fertility because it gives us more choices. A lot of couples seem to just fall into having children. They may want to have children and they may not. They may have the best motivation in the world or the worst. Or maybe no motivation at all. It simply happens. And for better or worse, they are parents.

Infertility, however, brings us face to face with our reproduction. Some of us will seize the opportunity that infertility gives us and choose to be childfree. As we explore our priorities, we will discover values other than having children, values that we can base our lives on. It's not that we would have been inadequate or unhappy parents, but that we found we could be happy without children. Our being infertile allowed us to make that choice.

And there are others whose infertility allows them to become adoptive parents. They have the opportunity to do something special, to share their lives with children who don't happen to share their genes. Being infertile gives them that opportunity, too. So adoption is another way of turning sour grapes into sweet grapes.

Now, you may be thinking that this perspective is ridiculously optimistic. If you are in the midst of an infertility crisis, it may be very difficult to see your infertility as anything but a cruel fate, and certainly not a special opportunity.

Remember, though, that we are talking about the real possibility for a happy ending to your infertility. We've learned that all loss brings with it the potential for gain. And the gain that infertility offers is the opportunity to live happily without children or to make an adopted family.

In this chapter we will explore the adoptive route to no longer being infertile. As we pointed out in the introduction, however, adoption is not as simple a word as it used to be. People have traditionally used *adoption* in its legal sense, describing the process in which a couple legally adopts a child of different birth parents. But as customs and technology have changed, adoption has begun to take on a broader psychological sense. It means claiming as your own a child who is not automatically yours by nature. Defined this way, adoption can also include donor insemination (DI), surrogacy, and embryo transplant, even though some of these forms of adoption require no legal process.

DI is a kind of adoption because a man claims as his own a child who shares the genes of his wife and another man, and a woman claims as her own a child who shares the genes of someone other than her husband. The reverse is true of surrogacy, which makes it a kind of adoption, too. Embryo transplantation is also a form of adoption because a woman bears and rears a child who shares the genes of neither herself nor her husband. Or a surrogate mother can be transplanted with the embryo from the genes of another woman and man who become the child's parents. Each of these cases requires some sort of adoption—of a child who isn't automatically yours by genes or by pregnancy.

And each of these cases requires a different set of priorities as a guide to your decision making. We are going to talk about these priorities within the overall framework of decision making that we described earlier in this book. In fact, we believe that the basic model we used to understand childfree can be applied very helpfully to adoption. The reason is that the paths to childfree and adoption are parallel. Both of them lead to a place where you can stop being infertile and start living again: they provide the means to transform infertility into opportunity and they are both life decisions that depend on a choice. First we will consider adoption as a way to stop being infertile. What we have learned from John Schneider about the possibility of transforming loss into gain we can apply to adoption. Then we will look at Rubin's three tasks of making a life decision as they relate specifically to choosing adoption.

However, our discussion of adoption in this chapter is by no means complete. Adoption is far too complex—technologically, legally, and psychologically—to be treated exhaustively here. But if you are interested in adoption, we suggest that you seek out more information to guide your choice. We have included a list of resources at the end of this book. These are certainly not all the sources available, but they will get you started in your search.

1. The Transformation from Infertility to Affirmation

In the Introduction to this book we distinguished between problems of childlessness and problems of infertility. Many infertile couples, though, don't make this distinction and assume that by solving the problem of their childlessness they will also solve the problem of the infertility. The experts say that this assumption is not necessarily valid; they suggest that before you adopt you should put your infertility behind you so that you can be what we call open to adoption. That is, you have reconciled yourself to not having a child who is automatically yours and can embrace a child who isn't. Open to adoption means that you are no longer infertile.

Susan and Elton Klibanoff, in *Let's Talk About Adoption*, describe this state of being open to adoption as coming to see adoption as *first* best. People who are still infertile (instead of no longer infertile) are likely to see adoption as second best. Such people, say the Klibanoffs, have distorted values that will not allow them to start off as good parents. "Instead of focusing on the meaning of a family, they are hung-up with the physical act of reproduction. If when they look at a child they adopt they see only the denial of biological children, it will be difficult for them to develop a healthy parent-child relationship."

But what is this state that the Klibanoffs and so many other adoption experts are talking about? Most books on adoption are very sketchy on what it means or how to achieve it.

We think that the best way to understand it is to return to John Schneider's model of grief we looked at in Chapter Three. His description of the transformation from acceptance to affirmation is what we call the transformation from being infertile to being open to adoption. And that is what affirmation is. When you can go beyond the acceptance of your infertility to the *affirmation* of it, you can turn the loss of infertility into a gain—the opportunity to build an adoptive family. At that point you are no longer gripped by the problem of your infertility. What you have left is the problem of your childlessness, which is a problem that adoption *can* solve.

When you can turn your infertility into opportunity, adoption is no longer second best. It is no longer simply a means of getting a child, any child. It is first best.

Joan McNamara describes this transformation as coming to see your infertility as a blessing:

> Of course, adoption may not have been considered until you discovered you could not have children biologically. But once you accepted your infertility, adoption can be a positive, first choice for having the children you want. If you can separate the desire to conceive children from the desire to raise children, adoption becomes a logical alternative. You might want to talk to some adoptive parents; many of those who couldn't produce children likely will tell you their infertility was a blessing in disguise because otherwise they might never have adopted the kids they now love as their own.

Open to adoption is the affirmation of your infertility, learning to see it as a blessing in disguise. It is no longer a curse but an opportunity. Just as in childfree, the transformation stage of grieving helps us to understand this process and offers us the hope that the loss of our fertility can be transformed into a gain.

2. Choice: Identifying and Removing Decision Blockers

We've made the case in this book that the way to

transform infertility into affirmation is by the process of making a life decision. The reason that we treat adoption as a life decision is that it is through the power of choice that we gain control over our lives and claim something as our own, which is what adoption really is. Our main discussion of life decisions is in Chapters Four and Five. In this section we are going to focus on Dr. Rubin's first task in making a life decision, looking for decision blockers that could keep you from seeing adoption as first best.

The problem is that you can't make a life decision about adoption if it is considered simply the next step in your infertility treatment. According to the Klibanoffs, many couples turn to adoption without really understanding what they are doing. "They think that since they have no choice but to adopt, how they feel about their adopted child won't matter. It is the only way for them to have children.

"But," the Klibanoffs insist, "they are wrong." We agree. It is only when a couple thinks of adoption as a choice that they can achieve the potential that comes with making a choice. Thinking of adoption as simply the next logical step suggests a tunnel vision that does not lend itself to making the decision to adopt. Adoption is not something you do when you feel like there is no other choice, not a last resort.

In fact, the word *adoption* itself is built on the concept of choice. In it we find the Latin words *optare*—"to choose, desire"—and *optio*—"free choice." Thus, Webster's dictionary says that to adopt means "to take by free choice into a close relationship previously not existing . . ." Adoption, then, is an *option*, a voluntary act. If you do not see adoption as a free choice, if you adopt a child out of a sense of obligation or guilt, then you are running counter to the spirit of the act. But if you can come to see adoption as a free choice, as first best, then you are ready to adopt.

However, many infertile couples are not yet at that point when they start thinking about adoption. There are decision blockers in the way. During home study for traditional adoption, a social worker will be looking for these decision blockers in order to gauge a couple's response to their infertility. There is a good reason for this. Social workers feel responsible for the children they place and take that responsibility very seriously.

They must try to find the best home possible, one in which a child will be first best, not a second-best substitution for a biological child. This same principle holds for other kinds of adoption as well.

The decision blockers we list here are motivations for adoption that may indicate that you have not yet accepted your infertility, that you don't yet see adoption as a choice. Our sources for these potential blockers are Joan McNamara, Susan and Elton Klibanoff, Jacqueline Plumez in *Successful Adoption*, Jeanne Duprau in *Adoption*, and Louise Raymond in *Adoption and After.*

You want to adopt:
—because you don't have a child and feel that adoption is the only option you have.
—because infertility has made you feel inadequate as a man or as a woman.
—because you are the one with the infertility problem and feel guilty about not being able to give your spouse a child.
—because your infertility makes you feel like a failure. (The problem is that an adopted child would always be a representation of that failure.)
—because you've heard of people getting pregnant after they have adopted and you hope that the same thing will happen to you.
—because you are ashamed of your infertility and think adoption could make you feel good about yourself again.
—because you want to give your spouse what he or she wants. (This can lead to a rejection of the child.)
—because you are bored with your life and believe that a child will make it more interesting.
—because you believe that you can "save" a child from some dreary institution. (McNamara says, "A child should not have to grow up feeling grateful or somehow inferior.")
—because you want to create a more secure home life.
—because you want a playmate for a child you already have.

—because you think that having a child will help you
fit in with other couples your age.

All these motivations tend to identify people whose
infertility still makes them feel incomplete. Without solving the
problem of their infertility, they may rush into adoption to find a
solution for their childlessness—a child, any child. Successful
adoption, however, demands that the prospective parents already
be complete, that they have a strong relationship *with or without*
children and want to share what they have with a child. Adoption
means accepting your adopted child into the family that you
have already made, not because it is an incomplete family but
because it is already a complete family.

And to be a complete family, a couple needs to have
solved the problem of their infertility. They cannot expect an
adopted child to do it for them. Being infertile means dwelling on
the loss of your fertility, seeing yourself as incomplete because of
it. In the terms of Schneider's model of grief, you are still
mourning that loss. Usually, all it takes is time for the mourning
to cease and you come to accept your loss. But some people might
get stuck in the mourning phase and need help getting out. If you
feel that way, try to get some counseling.

It is only when you have accepted your infertility that you
should seriously consider adoption. Acceptance means that you
are able to see adoption as it really is: a free choice, something
you can do because you want to, not because you feel like you
must.

3. Choice: Establishing your Priorities

When you have accepted your infertility and have come
to see adoption as a choice, then you can start to work on making
your choice. It is in the act of choosing that you embrace your
infertility as an opportunity, a transformation of your loss into
your gain. You are able to accept into your life a child who is not
automatically yours, not as a substitute but for herself. This is
being open to adoption.

As we learned in our earlier discussion of life decisions,
making a choice that is right for you means looking carefully at

your priorities, which are reflections of your values. This was Dr. Rubin's second task of making a life decision. It takes some work, of course, and much of that work is the communication that goes into making a mutual decision. We talked about the guidelines for crisis communication in Chapter Five.

Surely the best way to begin to establish your priorities is to gather data. You can't really make a choice if you don't have enough relevant information, relevant, that is, to your own needs and to your own infertility problems. Find books on traditional adoption, surrogacy, DI, and embryo transplant. A rich source of information is an infertility support group such as RESOLVE. Talk to your doctor about the opportunities for DI or embryo transplant in your area. Seek out people who are childfree and find out what their lives are like.

Gathering information and reporting on what you find is a good way of keeping the lines of communication open and of overcoming option blindness.

All this information will encourage you to start asking questions of yourself, questions that will lead you to discuss your values. For instance, Patricia Irwin Johnston, in *An Adoptor's Advocate*, looks at the various priorities that people have for their reproductive lives and how those priorities may influence their decisions. Anyone considering adoption ought to think about these priorities. Of course, every option is not available to every couple. There may be physical, emotional, or financial problems that limit your options. But the principle holds true: to make good decisions you must understand your priorities.

Some people, Johnston says, discover that what they value most in their reproductive lives is the continuation of their genetic structure, an addition to their family's bloodline. If this is what is important for you, then traditional adoption will be the least attractive alternative you face. You may find that surrogacy (if you are male) or DI (if you are female) will provide what you need. Or perhaps your dream is of a child who shares both of your genes, a child who embodies your relationship with each other. In this case, you might consider the transplantation of an embryo with both of your genes into a surrogate mother. This alternative is both medically and legally complicated, but it might be possible for you.

Other people value the control over their reproductive

lives that comes with family planning. For them, it is the loss of control over their fertility that has made infertility especially painful. If you feel this way, then perhaps traditional adoption, which turns control over to a caseworker and could surprise you with a baby at any time, is not for you. And perhaps surrogacy, too, as a few highly visible cases have shown, will not provide you with the control you desire. You will be better off finding another means of adoption that will give you that control.

Still others find that what they value in their reproductive lives are the physical and emotional satisfactions of pregnancy. A woman may see pregnancy as the fulfillment of her womanhood, something that joins her to other women past and future. It is an experience that only a woman can have. A man, too, may find great pride in his wife's pregnancy, in a way an emblem of his manhood. If you share these values, then you should look to adoptive methods that will allow you to enjoy a pregnancy, such as DI or adoptive embryo transplant, if they happen to be possible for you.

For many people, though, the greatest value is to parent a child, something that for them is one of the privileges and responsibilities of adulthood. If you see this as your major value, then you should strongly consider traditional adoption. But traditional adoption also demands a further exploration of your values. Here are some questions (from the same sources that gave us the decision blockers) that can spark some further conversation about the values that may help you to make a decision about traditional adoption.

1. Can you deal with information about the child's past? For instance, if you believe that women who have children out of wedlock are immoral, could you live with a child born out of wedlock?

2. How would you feel about having little or no information about your adoptive child? Would you feel comfortable with the mystery?

3. How would you feel about your adoptive child if you became pregnant later? How would you feel about your biological child?

4. Are you willing to accept a child who is older, of a different nationality or color? Could you be proud of him?

5. How willing are you to tolerate differences? How important is it for a child to be the image of yourself? Would you feel like you should mold a child into an image that looks like you?

6. Can you encourage talents, skills, and preferences that are very much different from your own?

When you are in the midst of a discussion about adoption, it is helpful to remember again that it is built on the root word for free choice. To give adoption a better chance of working, it should be a free choice for both members of the couple, something both of them should want to do. Better that way than to have just one member decide and the other be brought along by force or by apathy. It is by choosing that we claim something as our own. And this is what adoption means.

And, of course, choices are made on the basis of values, those we can rationally explain and justify and those that we just feel strongly about for reasons that we can't explain. Both kinds are valid. And there is room to compromise on values because some are held more strongly than others. But if you have trouble establishing your values or if you find that your values seem to clash with your spouse's, then seek out a counselor for help.

4. Choice: Committing Yourself to Your Decision

The third step in Rubin's process of making a life decision is to commit yourself to the decision you have made. If you decide to adopt, you should get to work. Committing yourself to a decision to adopt demands action. The enemy of this commitment is procrastination: you won't just find a child on your doorstep one day. If you choose traditional adoption, start calling adoption agencies and friends who have adopted that way and explore routes to independent adoption. If you choose surrogacy, find a lawyer who is an expert in that area and make an appointment. If DI or embryo transplant is your choice, ask your doctor about the arrangements that are required. Whatever you choose, it's important to get started on the fulfillment of your dream.

What if you decide that adoption is not for you? That's

okay. In the decision making process, the decision *not* to do something is as valuable as the decision *to* do something. Deciding not to adopt is not an admission of failure or of weakness. Plumez says that many people who would make good biological parents would not necessarily make good adoptive ones. What's important is that you have made a decision. If you have discovered that you are ambivalent about having children, then you should consider living childfree.

But what happens if even after making a decision and committing yourself to it, you cannot achieve your goal? Perhaps you have decided on a certain type of adoption and find that that alternative is closed to you. Or perhaps you decide to continue to try to have a biological child with no success. The important thing to do is to focus on what you have been able to achieve. All of your work together has made you stronger. All of your communication skills have given you a basis for solving most any problem that presents itself. The stress that has tested your marriage has given it the capacity to withstand even more stress. And with all that in your background you should have no trouble creating a childfree marriage, if that's what you choose.

5. Conclusion

Back in the introduction, we suggested that it is possible for you to stop being infertile even if you aren't fertile. Being infertile means that you define your life by the loss of your fertility, but being no longer infertile means that you define your life by the gain that can come from that loss. That gain, of course, may be found in becoming childfree or open to adoption.

In this chapter, we have discussed open to adoption by using the same model we applied to childfree—Schneider's concept of the transformation phase of grief and Rubin's treatment of making life decisions. The reason that this model works with both childfree and open to adoption is that it is so widely applicable to the losses and life decisions that we all face in our lives. In the loss of a job, of a best friend who has moved away, or of a spouse by divorce or death, there is the possibility for gain that can only come through grieving for that loss. And life decisions—such as whether or not to accept a promotion that requires a transfer, whether to take a volunteer position that will demand a lot of time, or how to take care of an aging relative—can be more effectively handled by using Rubin's three tasks.

So it's not that infertility is somehow a special case. Being infertile is only one of the major losses we will encounter as we live, and choosing to be no longer infertile is only one of the major life decisions. One bit of good news, though, is that we can learn a lot from this experience about how to deal with other losses and life decisions. Another bit of good news is that there is hope in these situations. Even when bad things happen to us, even when we don't know which way we should go, there is hope that we can work things out. We can turn loss into gain. We can make choices that reinstate our control over a troublesome situation.

As illustration of this good news is found in Janice Wheater Cowen's reflections on how being infertile affected her and her husband:

> All those hours of communication have built two people who know how to talk to each other and also know how important it is to take the time to talk with each other. Yes, our self-esteem was tremendously battered by our infertility, but it was also rebuilt as we learned to deal with the crisis as a couple and as individuals. We now see ourselves as crisis managers and as survivors . . . We know that we can allow ourselves to grieve and that we can handle the emotional impact of problems. We see ourselves as strong people who can work through difficulties. We have also learned how important it is to keep the various aspects of our lives in balance as we face different ages and stages. Our infertility helped us create a strong marriage unit that we use and enjoy every day of our lives.
>
> Perhaps what is most important about the way our infertility affects us in our middle age is that it created strong and sensitive individuals who had a chance early in life to discover what is really important to us as individuals and as a couple and how to nurture and maintain those things.

Being infertile brought the Cowens the opportunity to build an adoptive family. The struggle to become no longer infertile strengthened their marriage and gave them a solid foundation for living the rest of their lives. Loss can indeed lead to gain.

●

Epilogue
Mike's Turn

Jean got to begin the book by telling our story, so it's only fair that I get to have the last word.

I am concerned with the image of men I have been presented with as I have become involved in the infertility issue. At one RESOLVE chapter meeting that Jean and I were invited to, I was the only male there. Did the husbands of all those infertile women not care enough to attend the meeting? Perhaps they assumed that infertility is a woman's problem. Almost all the letters we have received were written by women, and many of them told painful stories of husbands who refused to talk about infertility or who decreed that adoption is out of the question and that's that, no need to consider it further. Now you might say this is only the woman's perspective of what happened, but whether you agree with the facts or not, the pain they describe is no less real.

Of course, not all men live up to this image, but there are enough who do to warrant my concern. But I am especially concerned because I see myself in that image.

I also used to be the strong and silent type. You know, the kind who confuses silence with profundity. Actually, I was usually just unsure of myself. I didn't know how to respond to issues that presented difficult choices, so I found it easier just to withdraw. Somehow the choices would be made for me by circumstance, or more often would be taken away altogether. Either way was more comfortable than having to deal with a problem.

But on the other hand, I was also a problem solver, particularly if it was someone else's problem. If, for instance, Jean would come home complaining about something that happened at the office, I would go into problem-solving mode.

"Okay," I would say, "let's look at this from another angle and see if we can find some solutions." Or, and this was even worse, "Sure it's a bad situation, but let's look at what you can learn from it." I never could understand why she would get so angry. I was only trying to help.

It took me a long time to learn that I really wasn't helping. Both of my strategies—silence and problem solving—were actually ways of keeping problems at arm's length. At that distance, I didn't have to feel them. I didn't have to be a part of the hurt and confusion that come with tough issues.

Infertility changed all that. I didn't want to admit it, but being infertile was difficult for me. Like most men, I had images of myself as a father—a good father—and I was seeing those images crushed. And besides, I felt like my masculinity was on the line. It was much easier to keep the problem at a distance by making it *Jean's* problem. I did what I was obliged to for the treatment and said all the right things, but it was still not my problem.

Two things helped me to open up. The first was attending a state-wide RESOLVE meeting in Indiana. Up to that point, I hadn't even met anyone else who was infertile. Though I didn't want to go, I found men there who were good role models, men who could talk about their infertility. The second thing was coming to understand what kind of pain Jean was in. She had to face pregnant women and babies every day at her practice and it was tearing her up. Somehow neither silence nor problem solving seemed to be the answer.

The answer, of course, was communication, which is a theme of this book. And I don't mean just addressing theoretical issues either. I mean talking about what hurts and why, and really listening to each other. I didn't have any answers handy, but it turns out that delivering answers isn't always what communication is all about. Communication grows out of the confusion of conflict within yourself or between yourself and another, and communication thrives on those differences. Confusion and disagreement are good when they lead to communication, and communication leads to strength and understanding. That's what I hadn't understood before because I had always tried to avoid confusion by patching up disagreements. Jean and I ended up having an extended conversation about our infertility, and it was out of that conversation that we eventually decided to live our lives childfree.

But perhaps the most important thing that came out of that extended conversation is that we learned to communicate. I learned that talking was a way of coming to understand. I learned that you don't have to know the answers before you open your mouth and that there is no shame in not having all the answers. Answers are only what you agree on and you have to communicate to find some agreement. And I learned that though problem solving is appropriate some of the time, other occasions require me to feel it, not to fix it. That sounds very feminine, doesn't it? But feeling is often much tougher than fixing, and usually far more helpful.

We were able to put these lessons to work right away in our next life crisis. As I finished up my doctoral degree, we knew that a big change was coming. I would have to find a job at another university, which was good for me but bad for Jean, who was very happy where we were. It was time to talk.

There was no right answer, so we had to negotiate every step of the way. I remember the evening we finally decided. After interviewing at a number of places, we narrowed our choice down to two, one she wanted and the other I wanted. After looking at every pertinent detail of each place, I finally saw that her choice was the best for us. It wasn't that she was right and I was wrong; instead, we had created an area of agreement: we didn't know if everything would work out at that place, but we did know that we had made the decision together and would do our best to make it work together.

The subject of this book is how to stop being infertile, but it is actually about the much larger issue of life skills. The lessons we have learned about the possibilities of transforming loss into gain, about making life decisions, and about communication can be applied to any major life stress. Our infertility, then, was not just an isolated event in our lives; it was one of the many life stresses that we will face.

The sad thing is that many people, especially men, fail to develop the life skills to deal with their infertility problem. This is sad because experts tell us that the way we, as a couple, handle this problem indicates how we will handle the other problems that life brings. What we are doing is laying a foundation for our future. If we can learn to open ourselves up to loss, we will be able to find the gain that loss offers. If we can learn how to make life decisions, we will be able to establish more control, which will give us greater satisfaction with our lives. And if we can learn to communicate with each other, we have forged links for a strong marriage.

I discovered how well I had learned these lessons when it came time for Jean and me to buy a house. We had set aside three days to visit our new hometown and find a house. Of course, buying a house is stressful in any circumstance, but doing it in an unfamiliar city under a three-day deadline is nightmare material. After two intense days during which houses seemed to swim past us and we were constantly negotiating with each other, we made an offer on one that we loved and the offer was accepted. At the victory dinner on the third day we thanked our heroic real estate agent for putting up with us under such trying conditions and she said to us, "Oh, it was my pleasure. You two disagree so well." I looked at Jean and said, "Yes, we do, don't we?"

Appendix
A Short Selection of Resources On Infertility Issues

General Resources

Andrews, Lori B. *New Conceptions: A Consumer's Guide to the Newest Infertility Treatment.* New York: St. Martin's Press, 1984.

Bellina, Joseph H., and Josleen Wilson. *You Can Have a Baby.* New York: Bantam Books, 1986.

Gold, Michael. *And Hannah Wept.* Philadelphia: Jewish Publication Society, 1988.

Henig, Robin Marantz. "New Hope for Troubled Couples." *Woman's Day* (May 22, 1984): 32-43.

Johnston, Patricia Irwin. *Understanding: A Guide to Impaired Fertility for Family and Friends.* Indianapolis, IN: Perspectives Press, 1983.

Menning, Barbara Eck. *Infertility: A Guide for the Childless Couple* (2nd edition). New York: Prentice Hall Press, 1988.

Pfeffer, Naomi, and Anne Woollett. *The Experience of Infertility.* London: Virago Press, 1983.

RESOLVE, Inc., 5 Water St., Arlington, MA 02174 (617)643-2424. This organization is a valuable resource for infertile people. There are over fifty local chapters of RESOLVE around the country, through which you can find information, counseling, and connections with other infertile people. Call or write the national headquarters for information about a chapter near you.

Salzer, Linda P. *Infertility: How Couples Can Cope.* Boston: G.K. Hall and Co., 1986.

Stigger, Judith A. *Coping with Infertility: A Guide for Couples, Families, and Counselors.* Minneapolis: Augsburg Publishing House, 1983.

Resources on Living Childfree

Bombardieri, Merle. "Childfree Decision-Making." (RESOLVE Factsheet) Arlington, MA: RESOLVE, Inc.

Burgwyn, Diana. *Marriage Without Children.* New York: Harper and Row, 1982.

Faux, Marian. *Childless by Choice: Choosing Childlessness in the 80's.* Garden City, NY: Anchor Press, 1984.

Lindner, Vicki. "Saying No to Motherhood." *New Woman* (April 1987): 57-62.

Smith, Anne I. "Childfree Living." Washington, D.C. RESOLVE *Newsletter,* May, 1985.

Sochor, Sonya. "Perspective: On Childfree Living." Indiana RESOLVE *Newsletter,* November, 1986. page 5.

Veevers, Jean E. "Voluntary Childlessness: A Critical Assessment of the Research." *Contemporary Families and Alternative Lifestyles.* Ed. Macklin and Rubin. Beverly Hills: Sage Publications, 1983.

Whelan, Elizabeth. *A Baby? Maybe.* New York: Bobbs-Merrill, 1975.

Wood, Lynne. Interviewed by Merle Bombardieri in "Childfree Living—The Road Not Taken: An Interview with Lynne Wood." RESOLVE Newsletter, September 1982. page 3.

Resources on Traditional Adoption

Bolles, Edmund Blair. *The Penguin Adoption Handbook.* New York: Penguin Books, 1984.

Canape, Charlene. *Adoption: Parenthood Without Pregnancy.* New York: Henry Holt, 1986.

DuPrau, Jeanne. *Adoption: The Facts, Feelings and Issues of a Double Heritage.* New York: Julian-Messner, 1981.

Gilman, Lois. *The Adoption Resource Book.* New York: Harper and Row, 1988.

Humphrey, Michael. *The Hostage Seekers: A Study of Childless and Adopting Couples.* New York: Humanities Press, 1969.

Johnston, Patricia Irwin. *An Adoptor's Advocate.* Indianapolis, IN: Perspectives Press, 1984.

Klibanoff, Susan, and Elton Klibanoff. *Let's Talk About Adoption.* Boston: Little, Brown, 1973.

McNamara, Joan. *The Adoption Advisor.* New York: Hawthorne Books, 1975.

Plumez, Jacqueline Hornor. *Successful Adoption.* New York: Harmony Books, 1987.

Raymond, Louise. *Adoption and After.* New York: Harper and Row, 1955.

Smith, Jerome, and Franklin Miroff. *You're Our Child: The Adoption Experience.* Washington, D.C.: Madison Books, 1987.

Resources on Donor Insemination

Curie-Cohen, Martin, *et al.*, "Current Practice of Artificial Insemination by Donor in the United States." *New England Journal of Medicine* (March 15, 1979): 585-590.

Noble, Elizabeth. *Having Your Baby by Donor Insemination: The Complete Resource Guide.* Boston: Houghton Mifflin, 1987.

Resources on Surrogate Motherhood

Keane, Noel P., with Dennis Breo. *The Surrogate Mother.* New York: Everest House, 1981.

Stern, Zev. "Surrogate Motherhood and Medical Alternatives for Childless Couples." *USA Today* (Periodical) (November, 1987): 70-71.

Resources on Decision Making

Cowen, Janice Wheater, and Carl Cowen. "When to Stop Treatment." A talk given at the Indiana RESOLVE symposium at Purdue University in 1983 and again at Ball State in 1986.

Rubin, Theodore Isaac. *Overcoming Indecisiveness: The Eight Stages of Effective Decisionmaking.* New York: Harper and Row, 1985.

---. *Reconciliations: Inner Peace in an Age of Anxiety.* New York: Viking Press, 1980.

Schneider, John. *Stress, Loss, and Grief: Understanding Their Origins and Growth Potential.* Baltimore: University Park Press, 1984.

Smedes, Lewis B. *Choices: Making Right Decisions in a Complex World.* San Francisco: Harper & Row, 1986.

Other Resources Used in This Book

Clapp, Diane. "Creative, Healing Muses." RESOLVE *Newsletter*, December, 1987. page 1.

Cowen, Janice Wheater. "Two Steps Ahead." RESOLVE *Newsletter*, September, 1987. pages 1-2.

Stern, Ellen Sue. "You're Pregnant . . . But Why? *Expecting* (Summer 1987): 18-24.

Van Regenmorter, The Rev. John. "Slow to Understand." RESOLVE *Newsletter*. December, 1986. page 4.

About the Authors

Jean Whitmore Carter is an obstetrician-gynecologist; Michael Carter is an English professor. They met in their final year as undergraduates at the University of North Carolina at Chapel Hill, where they earned two B.A.s, an M.A. and an M.D. They were married in Chapel Hill in the middle of all this education and later moved to Charleston, S.C., where they survived Jean's residency in OB-GYN. Next came Mike's turn, four years at West Lafayette, Indiana, earning a Ph.D. in English at Purdue University. It was during this time that Jean and Mike brought their infertility treatment to a conclusion by choosing to live childfree.

They have now settled in Raleigh, N.C., their home state. Jean is in private practice and Mike teaches at North Carolina State University. When not at work, they pursue a shared interest in early music as avid amateur musicians playing on reproductions of period instruments. Jean is also a dedicated quilter and still finds time for volunteer service, such as her membership on the national board of directors of RESOLVE, Inc.

Let Us Introduce Ourselves . . .

Perspectives Press is a narrowly focused publishing company. The materials we produce or distribute all speak to issues related to infertility, adoption or interim (foster) care. Our titles include . . .

Perspectives on a Grafted Tree

An Adoptor's Advocate

Understanding: A Guide to Impaired Fertility for Family and Friends

Our Baby: A Birth and Adoption Story

The Mulberry Bird: Story of an Adoption

The Miracle Seekers: An Anthology of Infertility

Real For Sure Sister

Filling In The Blanks: A Guided Look at Growing up Adopted

Our Child: Preparation for Parenting in Adoption—Instructors Guide

Sweet Grapes: How to Stop Being Infertile and Start Living Again

Where The Sun Kisses The Sea

Our purpose is to promote understanding of these issues and to educate and sensitize those personally experiencing these life situations, professionals who work in infertility and adoption, and the public at large. Perspectives Press titles are never duplicative. We seek out and publish materials that are currently unavailable through traditional sources.

Our authors have special credentials: they are people whose personal and professional lives provide an interwoven pattern for what they write. If **you** are writing about infertility or adoption, we invite you to contact us with a query letter and stamped, self-addressed envelope so that we can send you our writer's guidelines and help you determine whether your material might fit into our publishing scheme.

Our complete catalog and the fact sheet "Speaking Positively: An Information Sheet About Adoption Language" are available **free** from:

Perspectives Press
P.O. Box 90318
Indianapolis, IN 46290-0318
317/872-3055

DATE D

F

I

J

(

WOMEN'S HEALTH RESOURCE CENTRE
REGIONAL WOMEN'S HEALTH CENTRE
790 BAY STREET 8TH FLOOR
TORONTO ON M5G 1N9
416-351-3716 / 3717

WOMEN'S COLLEGE HOSPITAL

WOMEN'S HEALTH CENTRE

THE RESOURCE CENTRE

Aug 31/93